For Al:
For your friendship, years and
for your concern and support during the
past very difficult year.

With affection,
Dottie and Bill Bevan

The Mind Is Not the Heart

The Mind Is Not the Heart

Recollections of a Woman Physician

by Eva J. Salber

Duke University Press, Durham and London 1989

© 1989 Duke University Press
All rights reserved
Printed in the United States of America
on acid-free paper ∞
Library of Congress Cataloging-in-Publication Data
appears on the last printed page of this book.

Contents

Foreword   vii
Preface   ix
Acknowledgments   xv

Part One. South Africa
Becoming a Doctor   3
Sakkie and the Family   18
Port Elizabeth: My First Job   30
London: Marriage and Friends   39
Umtata: Rural Poverty   55
Cape Town: 1941   72
Durban: Health Center Practice   82
Cape Town: 1954   107
Emigrating   122

Part Two. Boston
Becoming a Housewife   133
Settling Down at Harvard   149
Transition   163
The Bracken Field Health Center   171

Part Three. North Carolina
Moving South: A New Beginning   211
Settling Down at Duke   226
Health Facilitators: Lay Advisers in
Community Health   239
Don't Send Me Flowers When I'm Dead   253

Afterword   271
Notes   275

Foreword

Dr. Salber does me great honor in inviting this short introduction to her superb collection of autobiographical essays.

As a wise and compassionate physician she has something important to say to the scientific and medical communities at a time when wisdom and compassion would serve each well.

Dr. Salber and I have been friends for almost ten years. We became acquainted during my term as Provost of Duke University. I had an opportunity then to review the manuscript of her last book *Don't Send Me Flowers When I'm Dead: Voices of Rural Elderly*, a study of the rural elderly in North Carolina told in the words of the people whom she was studying, and to recommend its publication to Duke University Press. I take special pride in the fact that the book has done extremely well as a Press offering.

Each of the present autobiographical essays is built around her reactions to apartheid in her native South Africa, her compassion for the poor and the underprivileged, and her observations about poverty, health-care delivery, and medicine in that country, Great Britain, and the United States. Each essay is beautifully and sensitively written and deals not only with the substance of the events covered, but also with the author's thought-provoking, sometimes disturbing, sometimes amusing, always touching, feelings as a physician and as a woman in what has traditionally been a male profession. The present volume chronicles a stimulating engagement with real world problems—very much a book of the head, it is also very much an affair of the heart.

Dr. Salber is a remarkable person—gentle, thoughtful, compassionate, but also tough-minded and strong. Her essays provide a great deal of insight into what it was like to grow up Jewish in South Africa, into the sociology and psychology of the health of the underclass and into the recent social history of South Africa, and the social history of the poor and elderly in an advanced democracy such as our own.

The great strength of the book is the personal picture it provides of a physician/scientist/humanist at work—how she designed her research studies and how she implemented her research decisions utilizing sensitive, richly varied innovative techniques.

What is particulary impressive is the role the author played as a mentor to her students, and especially moving is her ability to learn from others. This book will be valuable in seminars on women, work, and careers, and also as a supplement to courses on the methodology of public health or epidemiology. Those of us in the behavioral and social sciences in the health-related fields don't often have the opportunity to get into the heads of researchers as they design, implement, and revise their research projects. It is gratifying to observe that while Dr. Salber performed her work in three quite different settings, she always found a common operational thread in each locale.

My thanks to Dr. Salber for her work and for the opportunity she has provided me to read about it prior to publication.

William Bevan
Chicago, Illinois
September 26, 1988

Preface

The mind—is not the heart.
I may yet live, as I know others live,
To wish in vain to let go with the mind—
Of cares, at night, to sleep; but nothing tells me
That I need learn to let go with the heart.
—*Robert Frost*

My narrative reflects the interaction between my life as a woman physician and the lives of the people with whom I worked. Both in South Africa and America the communities absorbing my attention were poverty-stricken—most were black—and I portray the result of discriminatory forces on the health of these people. This interrelationship had a profound effect on me as a doctor and a woman, and I tell a good deal about my history, my feelings, and the growth of my awareness. Two social contexts, therefore, are important to my story—mine and that of the communities with which I worked—and I begin with my own development.

My background, place of birth, and upbringing, as well as my ongoing work experiences, influenced my outlook on my fellow countrymen and determined how I would see people, what jobs I would undertake and why, what I would learn from those I served, and how I would decide the proper nature of my role as physician. My book is a personal account, a case history, of the relationships between a particular doctor and the specific people she served. While I make no pretense of writing an academic exposition on social medicine, or a comparative history of the "two societies that are widely regarded as being the most pervasively racist in the world, South Africa and the United

States," [1] I hope my story may stimulate some students to explore these extremely important disciplines.

When I graduated from medical school in 1938—a white, undomesticated, ingenuous, South African doctor—I had only a beginning realization of the relevance of race to health. I was not a political activist. Nor was I a feminist. In my time and country a woman who chose to follow a profession did so knowing that her husband's career came before her own, that she would have to go with him when and wherever his work necessitated, and that the care of the children would remain primarily her obligation whether she worked or not.

Thinking back, I don't recall anything like a feminist movement or a call for equal rights for women during my years in South Africa. Harry and I took it for granted that I would work; we also wanted children, and we both accepted that their rearing would chiefly be my responsibility. I don't remember thinking of myself as a career woman, or as an academic, even at Harvard— I was a mother with an additional, important, and fulfilling role. The first time the word career was applied to me was when Harry told the children that he was going to North Carolina to be interviewed for a university post in Chapel Hill. Our daughter, just finishing her undergraduate studies—and caught up in the feminist movement—asked: "And what about Mom's career?"

Career women or not, all the working mothers I knew struggled with the conflicting demands of family and work. In my reminiscences I mention some of my personal conflicts because they are universal and because so many young women, particularly medical students, have asked me: "How did *you* do it?"

In my fifty years as a doctor I spent much of my time working among poor and underserved people in South Africa, Boston, and rural North Carolina. Despite the vast differences in locale and circumstances I found that people's basic values—regardless of skin color—were remarkably similar. In each place almost all of the people I knew loved their families, helped their neighbors, wanted and valued work, appreciated their independence, and hungered for respect and friendship. I saw, also, what happened to these people when faced with traumatic events beyond their power to control.

Wherever I witnessed crushing environmental, political, social, and economic forces destroying pride, I realized that self-esteem is essential to the health and dignity of people everywhere. In both countries I learned that being a community physician, in either urban or in rural settings, meant going way beyond the diagnosis and treatment of biological conditions in individuals.

My book is the story of what I witnessed and how my experiences shaped the direction of my work and my life.

I begin in South Africa where my husband and I were born, raised, and educated—Harry and I were classmates at the University of Cape Town medical school. We left our beloved country in 1956, our guilt at so doing never completely expiated, to save our four young children from the sins and oppressions of an increasingly severe apartheid system.

In my South African research I compared the growth of black, white, colored (mixed race), and Indian babies in their first year of life, recognizing that economics, social conditions, and culture largely determined the differences that I found, and in my clinical work I saw that health care can't be neatly packaged and separated from people's daily lives.

In the United States, aside from epidemiologic studies of smoking in schoolchildren and the possible role of lactation in the prevention of breast cancer, I focused on how race, poverty, and minimal education affected people's health and documented the serious variation in medical services available to different income groups. I realized that doctors were becoming too specialized and technical, tending to treat diseases rather than people who were ill, and knowing almost nothing of their patients' lives outside the hospital and clinic setting.

I enjoyed my research studies and felt they had importance, but what really satisfied me was both to investigate the causes of illness and to apply the knowledge gained. I had done this in the South African health centers where Harry and I had worked and again when I directed a family health center for women and children in a poor section of Boston. Later, in North Carolina I had the opportunity to assess the health status and health services of a rural community and to develop an original model for community health education using lay people as advisers. Later still, when I became closely attached to a number of rural elderly people who lived alone, I used both my pen and my voice to draw attention to their needs.

I was used to writing articles for medical journals, reporting on my work. But, important as it surely is, scientific writing is not the medium for expressing the conditions of people's lives nor for expressing emotions—theirs or mine. I felt this strongly when I worked in the Boston housing project and became connected with its residents. My journal articles were not enough—I could not translate into numbers "the feel of hunger." I tackled this dilemma in part by writing a book based on unstructured tape-recorded interviews with housing project residents.[2] Later, in North Carolina I had the same sense of limitation in scientific writing when I wanted to tell of the needs of elderly rural men and women. My statistical articles could not portray the feeling of aloneness—the widower's plea to "find me a wife." Again I used the tape recorder as my medium for conveying their messages,[3] but I was not completely satisfied.

When I wrote these two oral histories, I kept my own voice silent except for introducing and ending the books. At the time I argued that the stories of those I interviewed would be more powerful if uninterrupted by my comments, but now I wonder whether I was hiding behind those stories because I wasn't brave enough to bare my own feelings.

The present book is different. As I put my memories into a more or less orderly sequence and trace the development and pattern of my life, I become both the narrator and the subject of what is essentially a self-interview. Here I do reveal my emotions—my sympathy and antipathy, happiness and sorrow, confidence and anxiety. A compelling reason for this self-interview is that my experiences in South Africa, particularly in its health centers, were seminal to my development as a doctor and a person, and I had no tape recordings to fall back on. To write of South Africa I must use my memories.

And I have other reasons for writing this book. One is my deep regret at knowing so little about the early lives of my grand-parents and parents in Lithuania, the land of their birth, where they were set apart as aliens, just as black South Africans are in their country. I knew them in their family roles, but hardly as individuals with their own stories to tell of how it was when they were young. I want our grandchildren to know why we left South Africa, what it was like to grow up there (white, privi-leged, and unaware), and how our eyes were opened to the horrors of apartheid as our country deteriorated into a police state. I want them to understand why I am haunted by the words of Moagi, an eight-year-old schoolboy in Soweto, who wrote: "When I am old I would like to have a wife and two children a boy and a girl and a big house and two dogs and freedom."[4] And I want them to realize that it is easier still to not see the poverty and discrimination that exists today in our rich, hospit-able United States.

It was not until I had written a draft of this book that I was jolted into full awareness of how much being a doctor in neglected communities had come to mean to me; what deep satisfaction I had when my activities made a difference to people's lives. In a way that community work was an extension of family nurturance, but it was more than that, for as a practitioner of social medicine I was able to express my democratic ideals through my work. When I left each community, I felt a profound sense of loss and grief—deepened by the irretrievable loss of my homeland.

Because my South African exposure opened my eyes to the cruel doctrine—and terrible results—of apartheid, when I left my country I tried, whenever possible, to continue working with poor and displaced people, black and white. I tried to teach—for the most part privileged students—the concepts of public health and community medicine not as abstractions, but in relation to the people I knew.

In large part my book is about the "ordinary" people I knew

in South Africa and in the United States and the effect that they had on me. Most of us move in narrow circles with friends of our own social set, unless we happen to be fortunate enough to have jobs which bring us into contact with lives and circumstances that otherwise we would not know. Doctors have this good fortune and are thereby granted a special connection with people if they choose to take it.

I was faced once again with the problem of how to present my material. My own life could best be expressed through recording my memories. "It is the nature of old men and women to become their own confessors, poets, philosophers, apologists and storytellers."[5] But how should I depict the social context of the people I knew or worked with as a doctor? In the end I added some historical background to my personal observations and essential public health data on each racial group, emphasizing the inequalities in their social and health environment. But as with my first two books, I found the humanistic and literary perspective more telling than the statistical, using words rather than numbers in tables to illustrate how racial, political, moral, economic, and legal issues affected the lives, social state, and health of individuals and their communities.

Most of my working hours have been spent with men and women who made up for their lack of formal education by determination to make things better for their children. Some allowed me to be their confidante, to witness their hopes and despairs, their achievements and their failures, their joys and their sorrows. So I had the privilege of learning from two good sets of teachers— those who instructed me in academic knowledge and those who taught me about the harshness and humor of life. My second set of tutors taught me by unforgettable example, and I was drawn to them because of their patience, endurance, courage in adversity, generosity in helping others, and enjoyment of life despite its hardships. Accepting the beauty and the burden of their trust enlarged my own humanity and shaped me as a person and a doctor. For "what is knowledge/ Without the intrinsic mediation of the heart?"[6]

Acknowledgments

Over the several years spent on this project I have received advice, support, and encouragement from many people.

Four foundations—The Golden Family Foundation, The Josiah Charles Trent Memorial Foundation, The Mary Duke Biddle Foundation, and The Z. Smith Reynolds Foundation—provided generous financial assistance toward the expenses I incurred. I am sincerely grateful to them all.

At various times several individuals read portions or whole drafts of my manuscript and offered sound advice. For this my thanks go to Robert Coles, E. Harvey Estes, Tom Ferguson, Jack G. Goellner, Joe and Terry Graedon, and Iris Tillman Hill.

For their services in helping me obtain some of the photographs I wanted, I thank Ida Cooper and the Public Relations Department of the University of Cape Town, the News and Information Bureau and the university photographer, Anne Moran and the University of Cape Town Fund, and my friends Kathleen Crampton and Hedwig Rose. Catharine Carter photographed the South African painting which appears in the book and also enlarged family photographs. Whenever possible I have acknowledged each photographer individually; occasionally, however, no record was available. I deeply appreciate the insights and talents of the photographers whose pictures have added so much to the message of this book.

I could not have tackled the labor involved in rewriting the many drafts of the book had it not been for the skill, consideration, and patience of Sarah Vance who taught me—a beginner typist—how to use a word processor. I will always be grateful to Sarah for her unsparing helpfulness and dependability, especially during stressful times.

Inevitably, my family became involved. I mention in particular the assistance of my husband, Harry Phillips, our oldest son, David, and most of all our second son, Mark. From my earliest, faltering chapters until the final revisions, Mark voluntarily and patiently read my numerous versions of the manuscript and offered wise editorial comments. Isabel Huggan, a Canadian author of note—and my professional editor—added expert advice and gentle direction. My two editors also managed to reduce the girth of the book—painful to me but an advantage to my readers. There is no way I can thank either of them adequately.

I have left to the end the person to whom I owe the most. From the start William (Bill) Bevan saw merit in my project, steered me to sources of funding and possible publishers, and gave me his unfailing support and encouragement. Best of all he agreed to write the Foreword to my book. Simple thanks are inadequate. I can but hope my book will prove his efforts on my behalf were not in vain.

The book is dedicated with my love to my husband and our extended family—with special affection to our grandchildren—to our friend, Bill Bevan, and to the extraordinary "ordinary" people who taught me what it meant to be a doctor.

Part One. South Africa

South Africa is a country of black men, —and not of white men.

It has been so; it is so; and it will continue to be so.

—*Anthony Trollope*

Becoming a Doctor

As a doctor, immersed in each successive job, I seldom thought back to my early years in medical school. But a recent book honoring the late Professor Frank Forman, a revered clinician and teacher of the University of Cape Town (UCT),[1] stirred my memory, and I began to recall those early years, the reason I went to medical school, what it was like, what I learned, and the effect it had on me.

I don't remember thinking about studying medicine when I was at high school. As a child I often followed the lead of my older sister Polly, and when she went to the University of Cape Town to get a master's degree in English (with special emphasis on language), I was sure I would do the same, but with an emphasis on literature rather than language.

In those days, over fifty years ago, relatively few women went to university, since most of the jobs they took didn't need a university degree; those of us who did go were limited to a few fields. A very small number thought of engineering or law. A handful studied science and became anthropologists, chemists, botanists, bacteriologists, or pathologists, but most got Bachelor of Arts degrees in history or English and often became schoolteachers. Usually, even these women, once they got married, were expected to exchange their previous occupations for contented domesticity. I wanted marriage, children, *and* work, but accepted that my husband's career would take priority over mine.

My plans to study literature were changed by the economic recession in South Africa in the thirties and the practice at that time of hiring British-trained professors. My sister had great

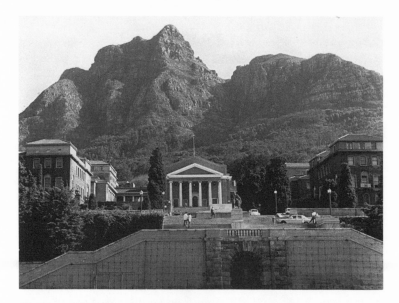

The heart of the University of Cape Town

difficulty getting a university job, and neither of us wanted to become schoolteachers. Rachel, a friend and neighbor and a little older than I, was studying medicine and was wildly enthusiastic. She kept telling me about the wonders of medical school and insisting it was the one and only career for me. Like most first generation immigrants, my parents were determined to give us the best possible education. I had taken the university track courses and done well at high school, so I didn't consider learning shorthand, typing, and bookkeeping in preparation for a future office job (which my younger sister was later forced to do for lack of money). Though Rachel's arguments were persuasive, I wasn't wholly convinced of the wisdom of becoming a doctor—but there seemed to be few alternatives. A few days before my seventeenth birthday in 1933, I enrolled in medical school—a six-year program begun after high school.

Looking back I'm struck by the ease and casualness with which I entered medical school. Once I'd decided to go there I didn't anticipate, or encounter, the slightest obstacle in being accepted.

Later I learned how sharp a contrast this was with women of my generation in the United States who had the greatest difficulty in getting into medical schools.[2]

First-year medical students were taught at the main university campus, together with other students in arts and sciences, but in their second year they were separated from others and attended the medical school, about a mile from the main campus. The university, built on the slopes of Devil's Peak, was splendidly landscaped and overlooked a grand view. The medical school campus, which included Groote Schuur Hospital (its new teaching institution), also had a lovely mountainous background, but its foreground was an industrial and poor residential area of Cape Town—making the hospital easily accessible to the people who needed medical services the most.

In June 1987 UCT celebrated the seventy-fifth birthday of its faculty of medicine. Before that time all South African physicians trained in Europe and very few women entered this essentially masculine field. As a student, I knew only two women doctors— both obstetrician-gynecologists—who practiced medicine privately in Cape Town. They wore plain, severely tailored suits— the recognized uniform of professional women at that time. Though standards had relaxed by the time I went to medical school, the masculine image of the professional woman faded slowly. When I was married and joined Harry in Ladysmith, Natal—his first army post in World War II—the other army wives disliked the idea of my coming. I learned later that they'd expected to meet an unattractive, mannish, blue-stocking type, dowdily dressed in an ill-fitting suit, unpleasant and difficult to get along with! I laughed when I recalled the women in the class immediately senior to mine, for they had been a particularly attractive group—good-looking, easy-going, well-dressed, and never short of dates.

I'd like to be able to report that, like Rachel, medicine fascinated me from the start, but that was not the case. Though I didn't analyze my feelings at the time, all through medical school I felt vaguely disconnected from the scene—an outsider looking in. Now, when I puzzle over the reasons for my detachment, I come up with three possibilities. Disappointed at not being able to study literature, I went on reading voraciously, spending more time on novels than on medical texts, and though I had a deep curiosity about people's lives, I had no overwhelming interest in disease. I could appreciate the hard work and often brilliance that went into the diagnosis of diseases—for which there was usually no treatment—but this predominantly intellectual task didn't excite me. Also, I may have been wary of becoming emotionally attached to yet more sick people—from childhood on I had developed a sense of responsibility for my family, stemming from my mother's frequent psychosomatic ailments and my father's losing battle against Parkinson's disease.

While not wholeheartedly enthusiastic about my studies, I was not unhappy. I always made friends easily and our learned professors, trained mostly in Scotland, were stimulating teachers. They stressed the biological and bacteriological causes of disease and the acquisition of diagnostic and prognostic skills, but therapy received little emphasis, perhaps because we had as yet so few effective drugs. (I was intrigued to learn, much later, how similar to ours was the content and the purpose of the American medical curriculum of that period—the same emphasis on the recognition of disease in biological terms, of being able to name the disease and foretell its outcome, the same disregard of therapy.) [3]

Our monocled professor of medicine (he lost an eye in World War I) was a therapeutic nihilist. He told us there were only five or six medicines that worked, and even these varied in their efficacy: there was morphine for pain, salicylates for acute rheumatic fever, quinine for malaria, colchicine for gout, emetine for amebiasis, and digitalis for heart disease. Even in our pharmacology/pharmacy course, where we made up standard household items such as castor-oil, the list of drugs we were given to study filled few pages.

As in Britain, the hospital wards were large, with beds in two long rows against the walls. Curtains were drawn around each bed for visual privacy during examination, but there was no way a patient's history could be taken without being overheard. Whites and coloreds were bedded in separate wards; though both groups were used for teaching, we saw mostly colored patients.[4] I think now what a good opportunity this would have been to show us the importance of social, economic, and political factors in disease, but I don't believe this aspect was ever stressed, though we were given a few lectures in public health by the Medical Officer of Health in Cape Town, dealing mostly with water supplies, sanitation, and food-borne diseases. Later, when I got away from the academic setting with its emphasis on individual patients, I began to think in terms of groups of people and the relationship between their living conditions and their illnesses. Only then did it dawn on me that I'd chosen a profession in which I could express my values through my work.

As in the British system, every course in our six-year curriculum was required—we had never heard of "electives." The entire class attended professorial lectures, but for lab and clinical work we were divided into small groups of six to eight students. As I recall, we women, placed in our own group and given a female body to dissect in anatomy, accepted these sexist arrangements without a thought. Even the female lecturer in botany addressed her remarks to the men. "Observation, gentlemen, please," was her frequent admonition. In a class of 100, twelve women entered medical school when I did, though only six of us made it straight through without losing a year or dropping out altogether. The first three years of basic scientific courses, particularly pathology, were notorious for weeding out the class—male or female. I hadn't learned physics or chemistry at high school, but I was a fast reader with a good memory—except for peoples' names—and didn't find examinations too trying. There was one notable exception. We were taught anatomy for a year and a half. The best memory couldn't cope with last-minute study of that mass of detailed material, and I came nearer to flunking anatomy than any other course in my life.

What I particularly remember about my days in medical school was how well behaved and disciplined we all were—a striking contrast to what I saw later in U.S. schools. The whole class stood when the professor entered and remained standing until he motioned us to sit down. If we were late for class, we didn't come in but wrote up the lecture later. We all took copious notes diligently and quietly, raised our hands to ask questions, addressed the professor as "Sir," and remained a respectful distance from him.

While I think they were all excellent teachers, some were more entertaining than others. The professor of anatomy, Matthew Drennan, was especially interested in physical anthropology and osteology. A Scotsman with an inimitable accent, he would shout, "Aaarrrchie, bring the bawns!" to the keeper of his museum, and in a moment, Archie, a pale, rather gaunt and silent man, would enter the room and without a word hand over the required specimens. In every lecture we waited eagerly for that moment, and each one of us tried in vain to imitate that unforgettable accent. At the beginning of the second year we were given a bag with a skull and a few bones in it to keep at home for study. I put my bag under my bed and forgot to mention it to Sakkie (our domestic helper). Poor Sakkie! Coming across the bag while sweeping, he looked inside, shrieked, paled, and almost fainted. After that I kept the bones in my dresser drawer. At least the bones didn't smell—unlike the dogfish I dissected in zoology. When I took that home to complete my exercise—working on a table in our garden—Sakkie wasn't at all bothered: he was used to cleaning fish.

The professor of pathology, Benjamin Ryrie, had an equally delightful accent, but no assistant like Archie. I didn't mind seeing the collection of specimens in the pathology museum nearly as much as I minded my first witnessing of a gruesome postmortem dissection. If performing postmortems were an integral part of being a pathologist, I decided that particular profession was not for me.

Charlie Saint, our distinguished professor of surgery, was a brilliant, humorous teacher and a merciless interrogator who made a fool of any student whom he picked on to present a case. I often stared at the floor to avoid catching his eye until he'd chosen that day's victim. In addition to his professional qualifications Saint had a reputation as a big game hunter. One day he gave us a lecture on bezoars, of which he had a fine collection. (Bezoars, I learned then, are concretions of matter found in the stomachs of some animals, hair being an essential ingredient of the mass.) Saint warned the women that girls who wore long pigtails, and who bit the ends, sometimes ended up with bezoars. Among the bezoars he showed us was a large one, the size of a coconut, found in the stomach of an elephant he'd hunted. I remember the first time I watched him doing an abdominal operation it didn't affect me nearly as badly as my first postmortem. The morgue had seemed to me a cold, grisly place, a laboratory of death, and the operating theater a miraculous place where those who slept on the table would wake after their ordeal, though I could hardly believe that the human body could withstand such assaults and survive. But I knew quite definitely that I wouldn't ever want to become a surgeon.

Professor Cuthbert Creighton, an Irishman trained in Dublin, taught us obstetrics and gynecology. We never knew what he'd say next to shock us. Abortion was illegal in South Africa (and still is), and Creighton would warn us about future temptations to perform this operation. Quite an actor, he'd tell us, dramatically, that people would come to us carrying bags of gold as payment for abortions. And, as dramatically, he'd warn us of the penalty of yielding to such enticements: Prison! Other advice had to do with being careful not to stay in hotels renowned as honeymoon spots. He himself, he said, had been called in many times when honeymooners got into sexual difficulties. His accounts were explicit, and we women prayed silently that we weren't blushing in front of him. The year we did obstetrics there were seven women in our group. He called us the "seven foolish virgins," eliciting a whispered response in my ear from our most sophisticated member: "How does he know?" (Or maybe it was, "Little does he know!") One of the best things

Creighton taught us was to have patience, to work with nature and not against it, not to rush into an instrumental delivery. "Put your hands in your pockets," he would tell us. With the male-dominant view of medicine then (which lingers still), he'd add, "Go play a round of golf." He knew we foolish virgins didn't play golf—his advice was directed to the young men in the class. But we learned his lesson of patience nonetheless.

Students were sent in small groups to the Peninsula Maternity Home (PMH), situated in District Six, to learn their practical midwifery. Each group lived there for a month, going to classes at the medical school during the day and doing midwifery at night. District Six had been home to much of Cape Town's urban, colored population for many generations, and it had a reputation for crime, drinking, and dagga (marijuana) smoking. We delivered women who were admitted to the PMH, and we also did home deliveries, supervised by the district nurses of the Home. When one of these nurses decided that a case of hers was suitable for a medical student trainee, she would dispatch the woman's husband to the PMH. The medical student next on the rota would be wakened to accompany the husband through the dark, deserted streets of the city. Many a time, walking those streets after midnight, I wondered what my mother would say if she could see me alone with a colored man for my guide. I never told her, but the PMH and its doctors and nurses were highly respected and certainly in those days a nurse's uniform or a white coat and a black doctor's bag protected the wearer. Nobody was ever harmed.

In my several memories of that month, two stand out most sharply. The first was my discovery that poor mothers and fathers shared their bed with their small children. I'd gone with a father to his house to do my first home delivery. The district nurse, very much in command, issued orders to the two of us. The husband was sent to fetch old newspapers which I was to place strategically under the mother to soak up her blood and fluid—I'd be cleaning up later. Then he was sent to bring a pail which I would use to dump the placenta in. Next he was ordered

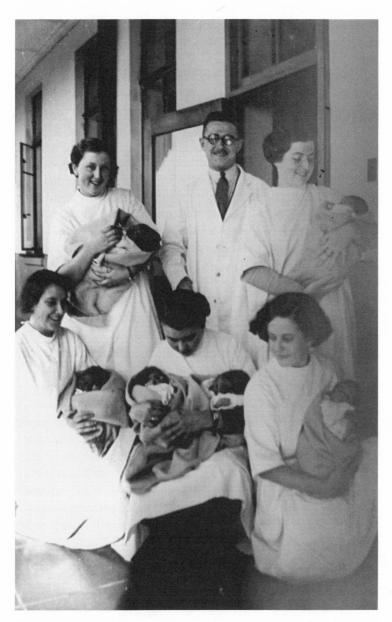

Proudly displaying our babies

to the kitchen to boil kettles of water to fill a couple of enamel basins. After that he was barred from the bedroom until the baby was born. I washed and dried my hands, examined the mother, timed her contractions, reported to the nurse, and responded to her instructions. We worked by candlelight, and none of us, including the mother, made much noise. Finally, I was allowed to hold the head, shoulders, and slippery body of the emerging baby. What a relief it was to hear the baby cry and see the mother smile. I tied and cut the cord—my hands awkward, but my heart at ease—bathed the infant and cleaned the mother. Every now and then I peeked at the curly heads and smooth, round, brown faces of the two older sisters sleeping peacefully in the bed at their mother's side. Many years later, when my own third baby was due, I asked my doctor to deliver me at home. He refused, saying "Where will you get the sterile sheets?" District Six flashed into my mind—sterile sheets for me, newsprint for my patients.

The second vivid memory is of constant weariness. Maybe those who practice midwifery and are accustomed to being at the beck and call of babies waiting to be born have little regard for students' need for rest and sleep. It's true that we were on a rotation schedule, but there were times when several deliveries were happening simultaneously at the PMH and in the district, requiring many students to attend. Sometimes *all* of us would be wakened at once. One night the bell clanged—the signal that we must all get up. The obstetric resident wanted to demonstrate a special patient. Each, in turn, was told to smell her breath. It was supposed to smell like "new-mown hay," an important diagnostic clue to uncontrolled diabetes. Drunk with fatigue, I couldn't recognize the scent. I don't know whether any of my colleagues could recognize it either, but all of us were indignant at being wakened. The resident could hardly be blamed for conscientiously doing his duty. All the same, though I've always found it hard to remember people's names, I've never forgotten the name of that particular resident, a definitely negative memory. I decided that delivering babies would strain normal family life—I would not be an obstetrician.

The professor for whom we had the greatest respect was Frank Forman. A South African, trained in Aberdeen, Scotland, he taught clinical medicine full-time almost from the inception of the medical school until his final retirement about fifty years later. Frankie, as everyone called him (though not to his face till well after graduation) excelled in bedside teaching. His meticulous history taking, his extraordinary powers of observation, his attention to detail, his vast experience, his phenomenal memory, and his encyclopedic knowledge were awe-inspiring. Almost invariably during a ward round Frankie would pause and remark: "In that very bed, about five years ago, we had a patient, Mr. Van der Merwe, with exactly the same symptoms as this man, except . . ." or some variant of this phrase. It's sometimes difficult to realize that in those days (before the tremendous growth in technology) Frankie could teach us, with perfect accuracy, that the medical history contributed 70 percent to the diagnosis of a case, the physical examination 20 percent, the lab and X-ray examination only 10 percent. (Today that order seems to be reversed.) Frankie's influence on the standard of excellence at UCT (clinical and behavioral) was immense, and many former students, now themselves distinguished, show clearly in their writings about him that they regarded him as their role model, their "beloved physician."

Besides his incredible store of knowledge and total dedication to his work, Frankie was loved for his honesty, his modesty, his gentleness, and his patience. He never put down a student or embarrassed him in front of others, and he always addressed patients with the same courtesy, kindness, and respect. Observing Frankie, I thought I' could be a physician, perhaps an academic.

Most of our clinical teaching took place at Groote Schuur Hospital. There, patients suffered the constant presence of students without complaint, and nobody on the staff discussed with us the trial it must have been when student after student would come to listen to a particular heart murmur or feel an enlarged liver or spleen or whatever. One story clearly shows the drawbacks (as well as the benefits) of being a patient in a teaching hospital. Certain patients with unusual conditions would be asked by staff to come to Groote Schuur to be shown to students. At a hematology clinic one day, the physician in charge smilingly told us he regretted the absence of a woman with Christmas disease, a rare hereditary blood disorder. She'd called him that morning to say she felt "too sick to come to the hospital!" There was no way to learn physical signs without examining the patients, and there were a lot of us, but all in all (and unlike the sometimes humiliating handling of the poor in large, impersonal hospital settings even today) I believe we treated patients kindly and with respect—following the example of teachers like Frankie.

Patients were accustomed also to being used as diagnostic puzzles at exam time, particularly for final exams. These examinations, for each subject, were divided into three parts and were grueling affairs. First we had a written test, lasting three hours and requiring essay-type answers. (No multiple-choice questions in those days.) Next would come the clinical tests, themselves divided into two sections. Section one, "long cases," would last an hour; the student would be expected to take a detailed history, do a careful physical examination, suggest what lab tests might be required, and come up with a differential diagnosis as well as the actual diagnosis of the "case." For the second section, "short cases," the student would be shown a series of people, on each of whom he could spend no more than ten minutes before recording the probable diagnosis. The third, and last exam, would be an oral grilling, conducted not only by one's own professor, but also by his opposite number at the only other medical school in South Africa at that time—the University of Witwatersrand in Johannesburg.

Notwithstanding our geographical isolation from the centers of learning in Europe and the United States, UCT's academic standards were high. And we learned important additional lessons which became apparent to us only by contrast many years later. For example, Frankie, as a full-time employee of UCT, was paid a very modest salary. He could have made a lot of money, for he was sought after widely as a consultant, but he never charged for his services. To him, and to many who followed his ideals, being a doctor meant a life of dedicated service, not a big bank account. His example strengthened my determination not to mix medicine with money—I would not enter private practice by choice.

Of all the events in my university life, the most important was meeting Harry. We'd met once before at a birthday party when we were about thirteen or fourteen. But, from about the age of twelve and up to my second year in medical school, I was partnered by my neighborhood boyfriend—a long-standing relationship difficult to break off. Having two young men who vied for my company in that second year of medical school certainly didn't help my studies, but I did enjoy the attention.

Harry often tells people that our romance flourished over the anatomy dissecting tables. His group occupied the table next to that of the women's group, and they were dissecting a male body. Walking from one table to the next, ostensibly in search of knowledge, made communication easy. I remember well the first time Harry telephoned me to invite me to a movie; I told my parents that the nicest boy in the class had asked me out.

Harry was more adventurous, self-assured, and pragmatic than I was. He knew what he wanted, made his decisions quickly, and accepted the consequences without regrets. I was more timid, less judgmental, more tolerant. I accepted his leadership willingly, though I did a fair amount of retrospective, silent soul-searching. Harry had a quick sense of humor and teased me from the start about my references to the "grown-ups" and my childlike belief that people told the truth. It took me a long time to learn when he was putting me on. More important than our differences were our similarities. Until we found each other in medical school, neither of us had met another person with whom we could be so frank and open. Neither one was overly ambitious, competitive, or materialistic, and intellectually we were on a par. Life was very different for me after I met Harry. Perhaps the very best part for both of us was that we became, and remained, each other's closest friend.

Harry and I talked endlessly and saw each other almost every evening. He would come to "work" with me, but we wouldn't get much done. With my good memory this didn't bother me too much, but Harry's grades, which had been very good until we began to spend so much time together, suffered. At times he worried that I spent too much time reading novels, instead of pathology or bacteriology. The evening before our pharmacology examination—we'd been told that we'd be tested on drug dosage—he went through the dosages of the hundred most important drugs on our list and made me repeat them to him. The next day, dosages fresh in my mind, I got high marks. Unfair as it was, I did better than Harry.

If I hadn't married Harry, I might have ended up pursuing an academic career in internal medicine. I liked that discipline best and scored well in the final exam, so that I likely could have landed one of the professorial internships in the second half of our first postgraduate year. But that period would have clashed with the time Harry had planned for me to join him in England to get married. As I made clear earlier, few, if any, women of my era put their own careers ahead of their husband's plans, and so, with suppressed ambivalence, I went to London in September 1939, rather than to Groote Schuur Hospital. But the war prevented Harry's plans for an extended stay in Britain, and we returned to South Africa within a year so he could enlist.

It's impossible to know what career patterns either of us might have had if not for the war. My first hospital job, in Port Elizabeth, started me on the path away from institutional and toward community medicine. Umtata opened our eyes to the horrendous problems of rural South African blacks. During military service in Egypt, Harry learned about the work of the Institute of Family and Community Health in Durban, which we joined after the war had ended. That exposure to social medicine the most telling of all our medical experiences and was strengthened by Harry's work with the Student Health and Welfare Organization at the University of Cape Town, and our knowledge of what a university could do to influence students toward understanding, compassion, and altruism. Participation in these activities in South Africa cemented the road we chose to follow—toward public health, community-oriented primary care, and social medicine. Looking back, I know we followed the right track.

Sakkie and the Family

Looking back, there are many ways I could now tell about the "colored" people of Cape Town—the racially mixed descendants of white men, the indigenous Khoi-Khoi, and captured slaves, Malay and African.[1]

Perhaps I should begin with the reminder that no legal color bar existed in the Cape before South Africa's four provinces joined together to form the Union of South Africa in 1910, after which "nonwhite" rights were steadily whittled away.[2] While we lived in Cape Town, colored and white families inhabited areas contiguous to or intermingled with those of whites; colored men served on provincial and city councils; schoolchildren were sent to separate schools after Union, but university education was not yet segregated; and disenfranchisement of colored men was not achieved until 1956.[3] More than South African blacks, the colored people have had a history and relationship to white society comparable to that of southern U.S. blacks.[4]

Social and health statistics tell their own story. Since 1900— when medical officers of health in Cape Town began to keep good records—they showed how much poorer and sicker coloreds were than whites, and how much higher were their infant and adult mortality rates.[5]

I could voice my opinion that to many white Capetonians the colored population is as integral and essential to the city and its life as their own presence. But, sadly, I must admit that just as I have quoted elsewhere that colored people have been called "God's stepchildren," so it is also true that they were and still are—often unconsciously, unthinkingly, but indubitably— treated as the stepchildren of the whites. Yet in 1966, when

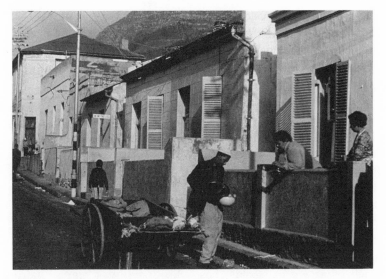

District Six before the Group Areas Act

colored people were removed from their homes in District Six, located in central Cape Town, under the outrageous Group Areas Act,[6] many whites expressed their deep anger with the government and refused to buy property there. These protests were so strong and prolonged that the President's Council, in 1981, recommended the return of District Six and one-fifth of the area has now been reproclaimed colored.[7]

But I didn't know all these facts when I was growing up and the danger of writing history backward is to assume knowledge to which I had no claim at the time. So I have chosen to illustrate the ambiguous position of the colored people of Cape Town by narrating the story of an individual whom I knew very well. One of the most vivid and influential figures of my childhood is a colored man whose first name is Isaac—Isak in Afrikaans, his mother tongue—but known to everyone as Sakkie.

I last saw Sakkie when I was sixty-seven and he told me he was seventy, but I'm sure he's more than three years older than me.

He seems to have been among us always, though he says he was ten when he first came to work for my parents. I believe while his mother was alive it was only part-time, but a few years later it became full-time. Staying with my family until both my parents died, he then worked for my younger sister until she moved into an apartment too small to justify such an arrangement. After that he worked a while for the local authority in the Division of Parks and Gardens, and then he found a less strenuous job cleaning toilets in a naval base. He is still with the navy, promoted to making the tea—much easier work but longer hours. Whatever else he does, on Saturday mornings he spends a few hours cleaning my sister's apartment. This is important to her, to my older sister who now lives in Israel, and to me, for we have regular news of him.

When Sakkie and I saw each other, we both cried and told each other we had colds. His wife, Rosie, was keeping fairly well, he said. One of their sons, who had smoked "dagga" in his teens, was now "married to the bottle"; one son-in-law was disabled and couldn't support his family; there were many grandchildren and Sakkie was still helping out. He had begun to receive a small old-age pension, but it was clearly insufficient in itself. The fact that he would have to go on working until he dropped was hard to take. Of course my sister and her husband in Cape Town look after him; my widowed sister in Israel and I send him money and clothes regularly, and he is in my will, but these are token payments for all he has done for us as a family—particularly for my father and mother. But what else to do?

How do I describe Sakkie? Medium height, about 5'8", weight about 160 pounds, regular features, big brown eyes, light brown complexion, short thick graying black hair, a ready smile. Does this tell much about him? Not really—to describe him takes much more than a sentence.

When young he had an irrepressible sense of fun; older, he stopped his pranks though he maintained a good sense of humor and enjoyment of life. One of my early childhood memories is of Sakkie baby-sitting for us when my parents were out. We wished they would go out more often. A natural actor, Sakkie would mimic our relatives—particularly two uncles and aunts who lived close by. We recognized their gait, their mode of speech, their mannerisms; gleefully we begged for more. I grew up in a home which continually sheltered "landsleit," people who came from the same hometown as my mother or father in Lithuania. Sometimes our guests were so distantly connected they fell into the category "Ferd fuss podkaveh ayn eynekul," (literally, a grandchild of the horse-shoe of the horse's hoof). These sojourners too were grist to Sakkie's mill. But his imitations, staged for our amusement, were never mean in tone. At times one of us became the target of his fun. My younger sister, who was born five years after me, as a child was plump and unhurried. Sakkie walked her to school, and, when the mood took him, would ring the doorbells on the way. By the time somebody answered the bell, Sakkie was faraway and my sister walking her fastest. Other times Sakkie would frighten us by suddenly deciding to lie down in the street between the tram rails while we implored him to get up while there was still time.

My grandmother who lived with us spoke to him in Yiddish. She also taught him "kashrut," the Jewish dietary laws. We had four sets of dishes and cutlery: a milk and a meat set for daily use and a separate meat and milk set for the eight days of Passover. It always took time for a new housemaid to learn the rules; grandmother "broke them in." However, if the error involved a small item, like placing a meat knife in the milk drawer, the item could be cleansed by burying it in the ground for three days. Grandmother was incensed one time when a new maid misused a big saucepan and wanted to fire her. "Don't worry, Bobbe," said Sakkie, "Varf aroys der top un begrob de shiksha!" (Don't worry, Grandmother, throw out the saucepan and bury the servant!)

They were really very good friends, but there were times when Sakkie exasperated Bobbe beyond endurance. One day, in great excitement, he came in to tell her about a disaster that had befallen Mrs. Stevien, a neighbor whom we saw every day standing on her stoop, her arms resting on the railings. Our trams had been replaced by trolley buses, and one bus-stop was outside Mrs. Stevien's door. Sakkie explained that Mrs. Stevien stood too near the path of the bus while waiting to board it, and the bus ran over her big toe. The ambulance had taken her to the hospital. A week later Grandmother saw Mrs. Stevien in her usual stance on the porch and inquired solicitously about her toe. When she learned that Sakkie had made up the story, Bobbe took a broom to him. Laughing, we watched her chasing him fruitlessly around the house; my grandmother had a wonderful store of Yiddish curses.

Sakkie was so clever it took us a long time to recognize that he was illiterate. When we at last urged night school upon him, he was too embarrassed to go. Ironically, my older sister and I were addicted to books and must somehow have taken reading for granted. One day we overheard Sakkie's conversation with a member of Jehovah's Witnesses who had come to the house to sell some literature. "Oh," sighed Sakkie, "I can't buy any more books. There are thousands of books in this house; I just don't have time to read them all."

Sakkie enjoyed dressing up and dancing. On New Year's Day he joined the "Coon Parade," an annual Mardi Gras put on by the colored population of Cape Town. But when I was in high school I discovered that he dressed up on other occasions in a fashion that might have got him into trouble in our more puritanical society. Not a homosexual, he seemed to have joined a transvestite group who wore long evening gowns for their Saturday night dances. I was too young and innocent to understand the significance of being a "moffie" (the Cape colored slang for homosexual), nor had I ever heard the word transvestite, but I knew the police arrested them and I knew, vaguely, that these men were bad company for Sakkie. I worried when I saw him with his friends sitting around our big kitchen table at night giggling and talking in high pitched feminine voices. And when he went out at night I worried that he'd be caught masquerading and be locked up. One evening I begged one of his friends to stop Sakkie from dressing up. The friend, who called himself "Dolly," was highly amused and informed me that he himself "was the leader of the lot."

Fortunately, Sakkie was a handsome young man. The girls liked him and called him often. After a while he deserted the transvestite group for girls as dancing partners. He seemed always to have at least two girls on a string at the same time, and I would hear him on the telephone giving convincing excuses to one girl for not taking her to a dance while winking at me and later confiding that he had taken another. He had a vivid imagination: I've heard him describe in minute detail parties we were supposed to have held in our house at which his services had been required and which had prevented him from taking Violet, or Sarah, or Annie to the promised dance. He elaborated on the meal he and my mother had prepared, the baking they'd done, the hours of tidying up later. I listened, laughed, and feared he'd be caught in his deceptions.

When Sakkie was in his thirties, we hired Rosie, a young, attractive maid who seduced him. Shamefacedly he informed my mother that he'd have to marry Rosie, and he entreated mother to be part of the wedding group. We hired a car (we didn't have one ourselves), decked it with white ribbons, and my mother escorted Sakkie to his church in District Six where, as I've mentioned earlier, most colored people had lived for generations (before the government declared it a white area). After the ceremony Sakkie returned to work. I asked how the wedding went. "This you call a wedding?" he questioned and went to sweep the kitchen floor. I stayed silent, sad at his self-entrapment, but unable to help him. Many years after their marriage Rosie developed epilepsy and couldn't work away from home. Sakkie looked after her well, and she had good medical care from a private practitioner and the Groote Schuur Hospital, the teaching hospital of the University of Cape Town Medical School. That hospital—known to Americans through Christian Barnard's heart transplant surgery—provided the main source of care for the colored population. (Sakkie once told me that when colored men got drunk on Friday nights, beat each other up, and were taken to Groote Schuur, they always folded their arms tightly across their chests to be sure they didn't end up as heart donors!)

I have made much of Sakkie's mischievousness, his playfulness, his pranks. All this is true, but his outstanding characteristic was his kindness. He was unquestionably the kindest person I have ever known, and with that kindness went a gentleness of spirit, a generosity and a loyalty to those for whom he took responsibility. He was for many years a wonderful nurse to my father, who was crippled by Parkinson's disease. Unfailingly patient and supportive, always understanding and sympathetic, Sakkie fed him, dressed him, walked him, turned him over in bed, never showing the least sign of irritability or anger.

I was very close to my father and did what I could for him, but Sakkie was his lifeline. I lived at home until graduation from medical school, then left home for my first residency hospital job, and later joined Harry in England, but I was home for my father's last year of life while Harry was serving in Egypt during World War II and I was studying for a public health degree; I was with my father the night he died.

However, it was Sakkie's presence, and his rocklike dependability, that gave the rest of us what freedom of movement we had. He cared for my father with complete devotion; my father, and indeed each one of us, loved him in return.

During my father's last years South Africa was going through a severe recession. We were always short of money, which added considerably to my father's anxieties, and I borrowed money from an uncle to pay tuition for my final six months of medical school. There was some money for Sakkie in the will though less than my father would have liked to give him. Recession ended after the war; my mother was moderately comfortable, and on her death Sakkie received a gift—her bedroom furniture and some money.

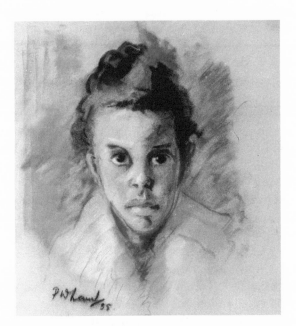

Lizzie

My mother, a warm, kind-hearted woman, was hospitable and generous almost to the point of irresponsibility. We cautioned her to wear two sets of underwear when she went out or she'd come home clad only in her dress. But she was also emotionally labile, suffering far more from a series of psychosomatic ailments than from her valvular heart condition which caused her untimely death at the age of sixty-two. Instead of psychotherapy, sedatives were prescribed and caused additional problems. We suffered alongside, but it was Sakkie's presence that lightened our load.

When my mother moved in with us in Cape Town, Sakkie came too. During that time we were visited by a Durban artist friend. Touched by Sakkie's cheerful service, Bill asked me what he should give Sakkie as a gift. I suggested a portrait of five-year-old Lizzie—Sakkie's first born. The preliminary sketch was my reward, and it eventually accompanied us to America. I see Lizzie's young face daily. Selfishly, I wish now that I'd asked Bill to paint Sakkie rather than his child, but the portrait is a source of great joy to Sakkie, as the sketch is to me, and Bill is dead.

I did no housework in South Africa. Few white women, even those without jobs, did. So it was difficult for Sakkie to imagine how I would fare in America with four young children and no household help. As I said, Sakkie couldn't write, Rosie could, and at least once a year she writes to us at his request. The letter that I reproduce here was, however, written by my younger sister from Sakkie's dictation, about five years after our arrival in Boston:

Dear Miss Avie [my nickname]:
I ask Miss Bapsie to write this letter for me to say thank you to Miss Avie for the money Miss Avie send me. Miss Avie will be please to know I pay the rent I owe and the groceries for when I was out sick. And I put some money in my post office savings book and the rest I buy Xmas presents for the family.

I get a red dress for Rosie in a new shop in Hanover Street. Miss Avie remember one day she give me a lift home and I show her where Mr. Max have his paint shop. Well Mr. Max he gone to Israel now and sell the shop and they sells dresses now. They was having a big sale before Xmas and they have such a crowd you can't imagine. I buy the dress for Rosie like I say but for Abie and Jannie I go to Ackermans and gets blazers, and for Lizzie I buy a blue dress with a lot of lace and a big sash. Miss Avie will remember Lizzie was so skinny she don't eat well, but she grow nice now and she get so excited when she see the dress she just clap her hands and jump for joy. And for Sophie I buy a big doll.

I cook a big turkey for Xmas dinner. Rosie have a fit the day before—just while she iron the new dress and she burn her hand so bad I call Dr. Cohen to the house. He bandage her and she couldn't do nothing all day. Rosie's mother spend the day with us like she do every Xmas. She is still alright, but getting old. She send remembrances to Miss Avie. Tante Nellie come to wish compliments of the season and she ask after Miss Avie. Her Peter he is going out with a bad girl and Peter spend a lot of money drinking instead of helping his mother with the rent. Poor Nellie she say it is God's will, but Peter is all she got and it look like she can't do much with him.

And Miss Avie will remember when Master die, Master say, "Sakkie if you have any trouble you speak to Miss Avie. Miss Avie will help you." So I write to Miss Avie to ask what should I do? Miss Avie remember Jannie he is going on for 14 years; he and Abie was both born on the same month only Jannie is two years later. Miss Avie will remember I get that council house in Factreton specially to get away from District Six and the skollies so my children can grow up decent and go to school and get a education and get a office job; not like me what can't read or write and was in service all my life. Miss Avie understand I don't say nothing against the old Master and the Missus. Master and Miss Fanny was always good to me so long as they live, and help me. Miss Avie know how I look after the Master all the years he is so sick and paralyse. And when I turn him over in bed to make him comfortable he say to me, "Sakkie you a good boy—God will bless you and your children." But Miss Avie I think God forget me.

The boys they don't do their learning right. Abie he leave school and work steady in a grocery shop all day on his bike delivering orders. He don't have the brains Miss Avie's boys has. My Jannie give me the big worry. A bad lot of peoples move in across the street and Jannie get pals with their children. I comes home one night and I smells something funny in the house. I asks Rosie but she say she don't know nothing and Miss Avie will remember Rosie like a

drop to drink herself. Jannie is asleep, but he smell of wine.
I wakes him up and I gives him a good hiding, but he don't
say he sorry. So then I watch him very close for a few weeks
and I don't hardly know how to tell Miss Avie I feel so
ashamed, but Jannie been smoking dagga. Miss Avie I beats
him and I beats him and it don't help. And the Master and
the Missus they is both dead and Miss Polly is far away in
Durban, and Miss Bapsie work every day in the shop and
Miss Avie is in America.

Miss Avie will remember how the Missus and Katy and
me cry when Miss Avie go to America and Katy say she
will never be a nanny no more for nobody's children. She
work in the kitchen in the cafe near the Parliament and
make the sandwiches. She like the work and they gives the
girls good food, but she complain of her feet. She go to the
Free Expenses [The Free Dispensary Clinic], but the doctor
say she is too heavy and Katy don't like to diet. She still
say she eat nothing just like when she work for Miss Avie
and she keep pieces of wurst and things in her apron pocket.

Well Miss Avie my legs was very bad. My lastic stocking
itched me terrible in the hot days so I takes it off for a few
days, but one of my various veins bursts and I gets a ulcer.
My Gott Miss Avie ek dink die verdomde ding will never
heal up. So I goes back to Groote Schuur Hospital to the
Outpatients and they gives me new stockings and new oint-
ments and tells me to stay home with my leg up. And Miss
Avie remember Miss Bapsie write to Miss Avie to tell her
and Miss Avie send the money for me and I know Miss
Fanny's family will always be good to me.

I so shamed for Jannie. We is colored people, but we is
honest and decent and no one smoke dagga in my family
before. I asks Miss Bapsie to make a appointment with the
Child Welfare for me and perhaps they will send Jannie to
a reform school. I doesn't want him to go with the bad
crowd; if he do one day he will go to jail. Ach Miss Avie,
Miss Avie's Bobbe say to me before she die, "Sakkie, look

after yourself a little, don't always think about your children. They won't bother with you when you is old." Bobbe she know what she is talking about, but I don't take notice when she say it.

And how is Miss Avie getting on? Miss Bapsie tell me before Miss Avie get the job at the University Miss Avie stay home and clean the house herself. How do Miss Avie manage? Miss Avie never clean nothing at home here, just always work in the clinics. I can't hardly believe Miss Avie scrub floors and wash dishes and clothes and polish floors and clean windows. And Miss Avie never learn to cook by our house. The Ou Missus and me we cooks all the time. Who show Miss Avie how to do the things? And who bring Miss Avie her tea in bed in the morning and get the bath ready? Miss Bapsie say no one. Isn't there servants in America? They say peoples is very rich there—how come they don't have no servants? And Master Harry he has a good job and the children is all at school and David at college. Katy cry when she get the letter from David and the snaps of all the children. She can't hardly believe her baby is so big now he go to school and can write and do figures like David say he can. So Miss Avie please write soon and give me good advice. And give my best to Master Harry and the children and Rosie send her love to the family while I remain

Your servant,
Sakkie

Port Elizabeth: My First Job

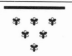

Harry and I had both graduated from the University of Cape Town Medical School in December 1938, and he had decided to go to Britain for his early hospital experiences, but because of my sick father I wanted my first job to be in South Africa. We settled that I would sign up for six months only and then join Harry in England where we'd get married and work for the next several years. So he sailed away, and I took a train to Port Elizabeth.

I don't remember too much about Port Elizabeth as a city—I hardly ever had time to visit it. It was, and I suppose still is, the second biggest city in the Cape Province—Cape Town being the largest. A major seaport on Algoa Bay in the southeastern region of South Africa, Port Elizabeth was founded in 1820 with the landing of 5000 British settlers—sent by Britain to reduce unemployment at home. A hundred years later Port Elizabeth had developed into a highly industrialized area—an important center of the automobile industry—needing and attracting landless laborers who were almost all black.

Because of its temperate climate and many fine beaches it was also a vacation city. One very well known tourist attraction was its snake park where several times a day an African, named Johannes, handled and displayed live poisonous snakes draped around his body. He was bitten several times, but the park had a large serum research and manufacturing section and help was always at hand. Johannes was certainly impressive in his skill and disregard of danger, but more beautiful than the snakes were the elephants of the Addo Game Reserve which I was fortunate to watch one night as they came to eat the citrus fruits scattered before them. That's about all I can remember of my own tourist activities—I don't even recall sunning on the beach.

As little as I knew about the town still less did I know about its inhabitants—particularly its black population.[1] In fact my knowledge of black people in general was scanty—learned mostly from distorted history textbooks at school that dealt with Africans in connection with events leading up to the many "Kaffir Wars." My six years of medical training had begun immediately after graduation from high school leaving me little opportunity for an education in more advanced history, anthropology, and sociology. Cape Town in those days had few black residents, the "nonwhites" there being almost all colored people. I began to learn about the black people of South Africa—at least about their illness patterns—in January 1939, when I started my first hospital job in Port Elizabeth.

The hospital, run by the provincial authority, had about 600 in-patient beds housing private (white) as well as public, indigent (nonwhite) patients, and a large out-patient department (OPD) used, it seemed exclusively, by black and colored people. There were no specialty clinics in OPD and no "honoraries" there, that is senior doctors who gave some of their time without pay as part of their hospital duties and privileges. I had been told that I would work in OPD every morning, followed by work in the emergency room (ER) every afternoon. This was to be my program for the first three months; after that I would be placed in the medical wards of the hospital. Unfortunately, no one wanted to take over OPD from me, and I was too new and unaggressive to complain, so I stayed seeing clinic patients for five months and finally had one month in the wards. Thinking back, I remember nothing of my time in the wards, but I remember some aspects of OPD very well.

When I began work on a Monday morning at nine o'clock, a tidal wave of sick humanity, an unending, overwhelming mass of patients, engulfed me and swept away my careful medical training in how to examine a patient. It had been drilled into me, over and over, how essential it was to take a detailed history (including a family sickness history) before doing a thorough physical examination and ordering essential laboratory tests. No one had ever told me what to do when faced with as many as 100 or more sick patients every morning and with emergency room duties starting at two o'clock.

I had taken over out-patient duty from the house officer (nicknamed Kappy) who had held the post before me, and he introduced me to the staff and procedures. Not the most energetic of individuals, Kappy usually began seeing patients at ten o'clock and, according to him, finished at noon. Patients were not given individual appointments, so most arrived very early in the vain hope of leaving early. Among other things that Kappy showed me were two dental instruments he used—one for the extraction of upper teeth, the other for lower teeth. I realized later that this was the single most valuable piece of information he gave me. I learned also that though I could admit patients who were too sick to be sent home this was not a simple matter, since beds were almost always filled to capacity and children's cots often housed two little ones placed end to end.

In a rather desperate effort to give my patients much needed attention, I began the clinic earlier and earlier and I skipped my lunch. I had three patients under review at all times: one at my desk responding to my very rapid history-taking, one in an adjoining room getting undressed preparatory to examination, the third undressed and lying on a couch ready to be examined. I relied heavily on the nurses, black and white (experienced and highly competent women), to repeat my hurried instructions, see that patients got their medicines, knew when to return—and I very quickly, almost instinctively, learned to recognize who was likely to die if sent home.

Once I'd learned to recognize rashes on black skins, I was happy to see people who had skin ailments—scabies and impetigo, for example, took little examination time. Dental caries could also be dealt with expeditiously. Each morning I saw about 15 to 20 people with horrendous decayed teeth needing extraction. I lined them up, injected novocain locally to save them from

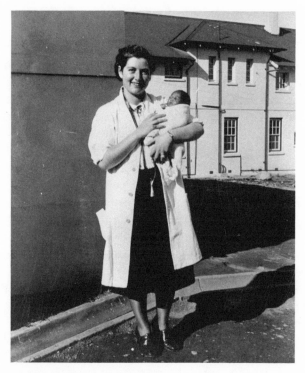

An irresistible baby softens a hard day

pain, and by the time I had injected the last one, the first was sufficiently anesthetized for me to pull the teeth. The two dental forceps worked surprisingly well. By law, sufferers from venereal disease and tuberculosis had to be reported to the City Health Department. Since we had no adequate treatment for people with these illnesses in the preantibiotic era, and the Health Department was responsible for tracing their contacts, I lightened this load by referring them to the appropriate agency.

I became tough in demanding in-patient admissions. On one occasion the sister (nurse) in charge of the pediatric ward weakened in the face of my insistence and admitted a sick, premature infant though her ward was absolutely full. She bedded the baby in a bureau drawer in her own office and cared for the infant personally.

But despite these shortcuts and stratagems, and no matter how early I began and how efficient I became, it was a constant struggle to get to the ER at the scheduled time. And, beyond seeing every patient, my time with each one was brief, superficial, and unsatisfactory—something was wrong with this kind of distorted medical care. Even worse was my realization that there was literally nothing I could do to better the poverty I saw, or to practice more than "Band-Aid" medicine.

Blacks lived in large numbers in a peri-urban, squatter, slum area for nonwhites adjoining a factory area called Korsten.[2] I had as yet no real understanding of their life situation, their poverty, their housing, and how these all affected their health, but somehow the word must have gotten out that I was sympathetic—certainly more so than Kappy. A new location—New Brighton—had recently been built by the municipality of Port Elizabeth with housing far superior to that of Korsten. A stream of mothers began to approach me, clutching their children all of whom were coughing. "Please doctor," each mother pleaded, "write a letter for me to take to the Superintendent of New Brighton. It is cold and damp in Korsten and my child is sick. I want a house in New Brighton." I wrote the letters for all who asked, recommending a change of housing on grounds of ill health. But, sadly some weeks after I first began to write these notes, the Superintendent replied that it was no use my going on writing to him—the houses were all taken.

It was, of course, absurd to put the newest recruit fresh from medical school into the most difficult job—one which called for experience, diagnostic skill, and the ability to recognize serious illness immediately. The job also cried out for knowledge of a different culture and the effect of discrimination, defeat, stark poverty, urbanization, and industrialization on African life—as well as physical and emotional stamina. Nothing I had learned in medical school had prepared me for this experience. Added to my problems was the fact that I was lonely without Harry and that all the rest of the house officers (medical residents), five in number, were men.

It didn't take me long to learn that Kappy had protested vehemently to the hospital director about my coming. He wanted no woman there; it would change their way of living, their freedom of expression, their manner of dress. One example he gave—only to his fellow workers—was that he would no longer be able to eat his peas with his knife. I should explain that the house officers all lived together in a specially provided house. Each of us had a bedroom, but the lounge and dining room were communal—meals were served in the house—and we shared two bathrooms.

One bathroom had no lock on it. The men forgot to tell me that the other bathroom had a peculiar drawback. Arriving sooty with coal dust from my long train ride, I took a bath. To my absolute horror, when I lifted out the bath plug, water began flooding the bathroom floor. As I tried to mop up this overflow with an inadequate bath towel I didn't see any humor in my situation; it seemed a rotten way to start my first job. The other bathroom could only be used if I was absolutely sure no one else was in the house. One day when I was convinced I was alone, I used the bathroom without the lock and lay happily soaking in hot water. Without warning the door suddenly opened and in came the senior house officer. Blink-blink-blink went his eyelids—he had a tic which became worse at times like this—as he stood and looked at me. I couldn't get out of the bath, and he seemed to be rooted to the floor. Neither of us ever again alluded to the incident, but even though it took a long time to empty a bath with only the tiniest portion of the plug lifted out of the hole, from then on I stuck to the defective bathroom.

Fortunately for me the young men soon began to think it might be quite pleasant to have a female around. After all I could be asked to make the evening tea and prepare the sandwiches. We grew to be good friends; they invited me to come along on

Sunday outings (three were on duty and three off each Sunday), and they became my tutors. I remember clearly one of them helping me to do my first circumcision. All had been at hospitals at least twelve months longer than I had. Soon after my six months had ended, I had to return as a court witness in two cases I had seen in the emergency room. The five men decided I must stay with them at the house, and one house officer whose family lived in Port Elizabeth went home to sleep so I could have his room. I was to join Harry in September, although war had been declared, but my housemates tried to talk me out of going. It was a minor triumph that Kappy was the most emphatic and protective of me—insisting that if Harry wanted to marry me, "he could jolly well come back." I felt I had acquired five older brothers.

All doctors, being ordinary human beings, have their own personal problems, big and small, which they are supposed to keep separate from their professional responsibilities, never allowing the one to affect the other—an obvious fantasy. In truth doctors have more than their fair share of emotional disturbances, divorce, suicide, drug abuse, and women, professionals or not, need the comforting presence of other women. Many a time I longed for a sympathetic woman friend, but fortunately I found I could trust my fellow house officers even though they were the wrong sex. A personal episode, involving close relatives and decidedly painful to me, convinced me of their ready support.

Not long before I came to Port Elizabeth my uncle, my father's brother-in-law, died. He had suffered for some time from congestive heart failure and during my final year as a medical student my aunt and cousins often called on me (unpaid of course) to sit with him when they went out. I did it willingly. My father was extremely worried about his financial circumstances during this time of economic depression in South Africa, but my uncle, who was fond of me, was a wealthy man. Without telling my parents I borrowed £55 from my uncle to pay my last term's university tuition fees, with our verbal understanding that

I would repay the money by degrees as I was able, after graduation. My uncle, who was in no hurry for the money, repeatedly urged me to take it as a gift, but I refused. His daughter, who handled his affairs during his illness and who wrote out the check, knew how he felt about the loan. But about two months after my uncle's death I got a formal, legal letter signed by his lawyer son-in-law telling me I owed £55 which I must pay so the estate could be settled. First I was bewildered, then upset and angry. How could they do this to me, the same person they had so often called on for help? And what should I do right now? My salary in Port Elizabeth was £12 a month, of which I sent half home. Harry was in England, correspondence took a long time, and I needed immediate counsel.

Reluctantly, I confided in my colleagues. Their indignation at my treatment was just what I needed. They came up with three alternative solutions to my problem: they would together pay my debt; I should simply ignore the letter; if I felt I had to repay the money, I should offer no more than five shillings a month so that the estate would have to wait years before final settlement. I rejected all three options but felt much better for being able to share my troubles and wrote to my parents.[3] In the end I was more strengthened by my friends' firm support than demeaned by the shabby behavior of my relatives.

After the first few weeks of adjustment, I was no longer unhappy in Port Elizabeth. I was far too busy to stay lonely; I had company when I needed it, and I even tried to play golf. It happened that one afternoon a man arrived in the emergency room with his beautiful red setter dog which had been bitten by a snake. I injected antivenom, the dog recovered, and his owner was very grateful. He was a golf professional and offered me some free golf lessons as a reward. But, after one or two lessons I proved to be so inept that I gave up the idea of ever mastering the game.

I had grown fond of my colleagues and of the nursing staff, and I admired and respected my patients for their stoicism and courage. Though I didn't feel that I was doing them much good,

I was learning a great deal and gaining self-confidence which I hoped might profit future patients. The sister in charge of emergency, with utmost tact, taught me how to stitch wounds professionally and helped me to develop my skills in minor surgery. We shared stories and laughed good-humoredly at the peculiarities of some of the older professionals. I remember her telling me about one doctor in private practice who had several contracts with factories to treat their workmen's compensation cases. He sent his patients with minor injuries to her in ER to do daily dressings. In those days we used gentian violet (blue) or acriflavine (yellow) solutions to avoid sepsis. With a smile sister told me, "He gets the money; I get the blue and yellow fingers."

With hindsight I see the Port Elizabeth period as my first awakening to the limits of clinical medicine as an applied biological science. I was deluged by patients coming to me for treatment of physical ailments, but whose cure lay in the reform of the political, economic, and social system. What they needed as physic was equality under the law, a sufficiency in wages, decent houses, education, and social security. I ask myself, what in that first job triggered my consciousness and began my awareness that for me medicine must basically be a social service? Without a doubt it was the impact of those mothers of Korsten. For they taught me, a fledgling doctor, to recognize the connection between their grueling poverty, their makeshift housing, and the illnesses of their children. And they asked me to *do* something about it.

On the train leaving Port Elizabeth my last thoughts were about its Horse Memorial. Erected by public subscription, it recognized the services of the very many horses which perished in the Anglo-Boer War of 1899–1902. In light of South African policies, which are responsible for places like Korsten, its irony is striking: "The greatness of a nation consists not as much in the number of its people or the extent of its territory as in the extent and justice of its compassion."

London: Marriage and Friends

My home until I married was in Tamboers Kloof, an old and unpretentious residential area of small, detached, brick and stucco houses, narrow steps, and neat little gardens facing onto the street, about a mile or two from the center of Cape Town. Trams went up and down our street every ten or fifteen minutes, the noise so much a part of our background it no longer impinged on our consciousness. Tamboers Kloof lay at the foot of Signal Hill, itself a continuation of Lion's Head which flanked Table Mountain. Just as the mountain was an indelible part of our existence so was the twelve o'clock signal fired each noon from the top of Signal Hill. At the sound of the cannon everyone in Cape Town (at least those who owned watches) stopped dead in their tracks and adjusted their timepieces.

Tamboers Kloof was, I think, an all white suburb, but it was not something I heard discussed as a child. We were more conscious that we were Jews in a predominantly Afrikaner area, for my parents' friends were Jews as were my playmates. We knew my father had left Lithuania to avoid being dragooned into the Russian army to serve in the Russo-Japanese War, and we, in common with all immigrant Jews, sheltered others throughout the years. All my father's siblings lived close by, except for the oldest brother. He had been the one to bring them to South Africa, but later he returned to Lithuania and so to his death in the Holocaust. My grandmother told me enough about pogroms to shock me into an awareness of religious persecution. My father taught me about Jewish life, culture, ethics, and poverty in the old country by reading to me in Yiddish from his large collection of Yiddish classics. My mother taught me, by example, that Jews cared for and shared with those in need.

Harry grew up in Wynberg, eight miles to the south of Cape Town. His parents took a more circuitous route to South Africa, his father having left Russia at the age of twelve, taking a brother of ten in tow, to seek a living for the family in the sweatshops of London. As a young adventurous man of nineteen he took passage to the Cape, liked what he saw, and returned there in 1904 with his wife. He, along with his siblings, also tried life in America, but unlike those brothers and sisters who settled there, he and his wife settled in South Africa. Harry's parents were exposed to class struggle, to the anarchist and socialist movements at the end of the nineteenth century, and to secular rather than religious ethical ideas. Though they chose not to attend services, they paid their dues to the local synagogue. They, like my parents, mixed almost solely with other Jewish families in Cape Town, and, like my own, Harry's companions at school were almost all Jews.

Jews were the main white immigrant group in South Africa around the turn of the century and to a large extent were isolated socially from the mainstream of society. They came as uneducated (except in their own religious culture), poor strangers speaking a broken English and an even more broken Afrikaans. Untutored as they were, they turned their hands to occupations far removed from their lives in the *shtetls* of Eastern Europe. My father, for example, became a buyer of livestock for the wholesale meat business he and his brothers owned, and once proudly sent home a clipping describing a cattle show to which he'd been appointed judge. Jews have been a success story in South Africa, but even today number only 100,000 to 150,000 people.

On the whole, because of their own experience of persecution, Jews have been a liberal group in South Africa. I'm uncertain at what age Harry and I began to question racial policies. We were in part blinded because colored people in Cape Town suffered far less discrimination than did blacks elsewhere in South Africa. But we must have been quite young, for in college we discovered that each of us had chosen to expound the virtues of socialism in our high schools' respective debating societies. Though it was mainly an intellectual questioning—we were not political activists—it shaped our social attitudes. I recall, also, that my sister's best friend at college was a strikingly beautiful young colored woman who often visited.

Harry and I entered medical school at the same time, he with a much more positive approach to being a doctor. By our second year of school we knew we'd eventually get married, but we'd have to postpone it until we were no longer students, for in those days marriages between students was almost unheard of. A husband was supposed to be able to support his wife before he married her, so we had to wait until we had graduated even to become engaged, and World War II was declared three weeks before I was due to leave South Africa. Still, at twenty-three danger seemed remote and marriage more important than the hazards of war.

My grandmother was a tough woman not given to tears or sentiment, except when she read the romantic serials in her weekly Yiddish paper. But we were very fond of each other, she often saying, "First God and then you," and she was troubled by our plans for a civil marriage. In her eyes marriage in a registry office was not ordained for Jewish brides, and in the fashion of orthodox Jews who directly address their Almighty, she made a personal contract with Him. My knowledge of Yiddish isn't good enough to repeat her actual words, but she was confident of God's blessing and protection from German warships if I'd promise to get married in traditional Jewish fashion in a synagogue. She assured me my father wouldn't die while I was gone if only I heeded her bidding. I gave my promise and kept it (after slight delay).

Nestling at the foot of Table Mountain, with its tablecloth of cloud, Cape Town still is to me (and to most South Africans) the most beautiful city in the world. The mountain rises a thousand meters high in a sheer mass from Table Bay. It can be seen as a backdrop to the city wherever one stands, but nowhere is its magnificence more apparent than from the sea. So I remained at the ship's rail, waving to my well-wishers and watching the city of the mountain recede until I could see it no longer.

Wide awake that first night on the ship, I lay thinking of my recent conversation with Bertie, Harry's older brother, and my indignant but suppressed reactions to his admonitions. "Do you really think it's right for you to go now?" Bertie questioned. Thinking he meant the physical danger to me, I made light of it. But he didn't mean that at all. Since Harry and I had been virtually tied together for at least five of our six years of medical school, he said that I was about to deprive Harry of the chance "to sow his wild oats!" That I would have preferred not to leave home at that particular juncture, that it would have been easier on me if Harry had returned to get married rather than have me join him, was irrelevant to Bertie. And, of course, with his complete acceptance of the customary double standard, he never even thought to talk of the possible liberating effect of a delayed marriage on *my* wild oats. Bertie then went on to read me a solemn homily on the needs of young men and made me feel selfish and guiltily possessive. Knowing exactly what Harry would say when I told him this story kept me outwardly calm. But all I can remember replying to Bertie was my cowardly, "I'll tell Harry what you said and ask him if he would like to postpone our wedding."

It was a strange journey of two weeks. Only a handful of passengers, nineteen in all, were on board: men returning to enlist, wives to rejoin husbands, Britishers going home. I was an alien to the group. Since there were hardly any women on the ship, I spent a fair amount of time with a young, good-looking, expensively dressed blonde who was returning to her fiancé. She borrowed half of my total sum of £45, which I had great difficulty in reclaiming. I must have spoken of my work in Port Elizabeth and the plight of the Africans I had treated, for she thought I wouldn't mind sharing what I had with her since she took me to be a socialist.

Most of the passengers spent inordinate amounts of time in the ship's bar—my introduction to the British love of pubs. We all listened closely to the frequent news broadcasts, particularly to reports of armed raiders close by. Unescorted, relying on speed to outrun the enemy, we showed no lights at night. By instruction of the captain each of us readied a small emergency suitcase to take along if ordered to abandon ship. Mine held a skirt and sweater, a change of underclothes, and my packet of love letters.

Finally, Southampton and a greeting of gray cheerless skies and fine drizzle. A deep, sinking feeling of disappointment mixed with panic came over me. I expected to see a loving fiancé at the docks, but there was no one to meet the ship. I didn't know Harry's London address—he had moved about the time I boarded ship—and I had no idea how to reach him. Should I go to the police for help? While I mulled over what I should do, to my enormous relief the purser approached me with a letter bearing a familiar, reassuring handwriting. The Admiralty wouldn't allow ships' arrival dates to be published, so Harry had been in touch daily with the Union Castle Steamship company who advised him to write a letter to the ship to await its arrival. The letter held a welcome which cheered me considerably and several contingency instructions. I was to send a telegram to his Paddington address (enclosed in the letter), and he'd meet the boat train at Waterloo Station. If by chance we missed each other (I wondered how that would be possible but soon enough found out), I was to take a cab to the Mount Royal Hotel in Marble Arch and telephone him from there. He spelled out one particularly thoughtful detail: the call would cost two pence, he wrote, but if there was no reply I was to press button B and I'd get my money back. Grateful for those details, I felt that with luck we'd see each other in a couple of hours, and life could begin again. Maybe it would even stop raining.

Southampton Docks were grimy, ugly, desolate. The fall air was thick and cold. The houses I passed on the train ride to London seemed monotonously shabby; coal dust smudged the passengers and streaked the wet train windows—my sooty face matching the passing gloomy scene. It dawned on me that I was hungry: I had not eaten since seven that morning—we had docked at two; in my excitement I had skipped lunch. What a contrast to the scene I had left two weeks earlier: mountain beauty, blue sea, bright sunshine, warmth, fresh air.

It must have been late afternoon when the train reached Waterloo Station, and it was already dark. Waterloo Station had a glass roof and hadn't yet been prepared for blackout. No lights were turned on, and I knew Harry and I would never find each other there. I kept approaching men to see if one of them might be Harry, but stopped when I realized that my actions could be misinterpreted. What to do next? The instructions had been to go to a hotel in Marble Arch. I had no idea where Marble Arch was, nor could I see anything but blackness as I peered through the windows of the taxi. It rained steadily. My hat dropped into the wet gutter as I got out of the cab, and I was relieved to have one less object to look after—I hated hats anyhow—but I was getting bedraggled.

Clutching my heavy suitcase in one hand, my emergency suitcase and pocketbook in the other, I climbed a flight of stairs to the reception desk and asked for Harry. He wasn't there, and there was no message. For the next hour, at regular five minute intervals, I telephoned his number in Paddington, got no reply, pressed button B, and got my two pennies back. At long last Harry answered the telephone. He'd been in touch with the shipping company the previous day to ask if the ship might be arriving the next day, had been told it would not, and had gone to the movies with a friend, and then to supper with him. At the restaurant he called his landlady to check for possible messages and was told that a telegram had come. Knowing he couldn't get to Waterloo in time to meet me, Harry rushed back to Paddington to wait for my call. (His first hospital job had been in the north of England at Stockton-on-Tees, but he'd finished his contract and come to London well ahead of my expected arrival, staying in a small rooming house in Paddington.) Wanting to receive me in style, he'd booked accommodation for our first few days together in a hotel in Marble Arch, in London's West End.

I sat waiting in the hotel vestibule, my chair placed so that I could see anyone who came up the stairs. My appearance was far from bridelike—my dress was wrinkled, my hair disheveled, my suitcase battered. At nine that night my spirits soared and my face lit up as I saw Harry running up that staircase. He told me he had run all the way but was forced to stop at one busy intersection when an old lady asked him to help her across the street. At first he pretended not to hear her and began to cross, then went back to help her before starting to run again. He spoke to the receptionist, disposed of my luggage, and took me to the nearest cafe for tea and a sandwich. Miraculously it *had* stopped raining.

The morning after my arrival we went to the nearest registry office to get married; we had bought the wedding ring in South Africa. But the clerk explained that Marble Arch was in a different borough; if Harry had not moved from Paddington, we could have gotten married there, but having moved, we must give two weeks notice of intent to marry. Two weeks later we returned, with the date October 31, 1939, stamped inside the ring, only to be told that now we could apply for a special license and be married twenty-four hours later! We again notified our closest friends—Basil, whom Harry had met on the voyage to Britain, and Philip and Ben, whom he had known slightly at home and who had become good friends now in London. Ben couldn't come, but Basil and Philip would be our witnesses. We should have known better; Philip was always late for appointments.

After waiting for Philip in the Marylebone Town Hall until we could wait no longer, Harry went outside and offered a passerby half a crown to act as witness. During the ceremony Philip crept in sheepishly, chagrined at being displaced by a stranger. To celebrate our wedding we took Philip, Ben, and Basil to lunch in a Spanish restaurant. We liked Spanish food but didn't want to support any Franco sympathizer, so we carefully checked the political affiliations of several restaurant owners. The republican owner of the place we chose joined our celebration by demonstrating the use of the Spanish flagon; so adept was he that he kept a lighted cigarette in one corner of his mouth while pouring wine into the other corner without spilling a drop. I applauded those brave enough to follow his example, but I had too few dresses to take such a chance and meekly asked for a glass. Before we left our host toasted us in macho Spanish style: "Salud, pesetas, y fuerza en la bragueta!"

Gasoline was rationed, but doctors could get a small allowance. Harry had bought an old secondhand car in Stockton and had saved some coupons. For a week we honeymooned in the beautiful English countryside, our personal life far removed from the war around us. We were young and in love, and I was free of responsibility—no patients or parents to worry about. I was intoxicated with my freedom.

Returning to reality after our dream week, we had to become more practical, sell the car, find a less expensive place to live, and look for jobs. So many people had left London for the safety of the countryside that it was easy to find suitable accommodation in "classy" areas. We moved into a flat in Welbeck Street, very near Harley Street, for only two guineas a week. Located on the fourth floor—no elevator—we climbed the stairs sedately, except that when we reached the third floor landing Harry always pinched me to make me squeal in order to shock the two elderly, spinster sisters who lived in that genteel building. The owner of the flats lived on the ground floor in a spacious and expensive flat, but most of the rooms in the building were vacant. It was cold—shillings for the gas fire didn't last long—and sometimes I'd smoke one of Harry's pipes, cradling my hands around the bowl for warmth. But even two guineas a week was more than we could afford for long, and I asked the manager if the rent could be lowered. He reported back that it was not possible for "it would lower the tone of the street!" We obviously didn't belong in Welbeck Street and moved to a cheaper area.

What seemed to us the most realistic and sensible pattern of our future movements was soon established. Harry must find a job first, then I would know which of the advertised jobs to apply for so I could be as near to him as possible. When he accepted a job at the Sutton and Cheam Hospital in Surrey, I enrolled for a term at the Postgraduate School in Hammersmith where our teachers were men whose names adorned the textbooks we used. Many of the students were friendly expatriates with an irreverent sense of humor about British hallowed traditions. I remember hearing a ditty which poked fun at the king's physician: Lord Dawson of Penn / has killed many men / That's why we sing / God save the King.

In those days medical house officers (and nursing) staff were required to live in accommodation provided by the hospital—easing access to the wards for night and weekend duty. Like provision for live-in maids, board and lodging on the premises made up a large part of the salary (in kind) and was never questioned. And, as with domestic workers, such provision was often spartan. Because medical house officers were treated as being single, regardless of their marital status, I was not allowed to live in the Sutton hospital.

Where I would live till I found employment worried us a lot. Because I have no sense of direction, Harry gave me daily geography lessons on London streets. I could answer his quizzes about "What streets come out of Cambridge Circus?" and so on because I had a good memory, but it meant nothing to me visually. One time Harry left me about a mile from our lodging, carefully explaining how I was to get back; almost two hours later he was about to go to the police station when I arrived. I had gone on the correct street but turned right instead of left.

I ended up living in Dollis Hill, in North London, with some distant relatives who had come on hard times. The husband had a modestly successful fruit importing business until the war destroyed it. My twenty-five shillings a week rent and board helped them out. But it was a *very* cold winter, and the house was very poorly heated—coal was rationed and expensive. When Harry came to spend the weekend, I watched him turning blue as he undressed! He begged me to leave, but I felt I couldn't—by then I knew they depended on my rent money.

When I first came to live in Dollis Hill, I asked politely when the family bathed so that I could fit in with their routine, but I soon found out that they were far too sensible to take daily baths in that freezing bathroom. I was warm only when I was covered up to my neck. The worst time came when the pipes froze, and we had no water at all except what we carried in buckets from the city mains in the street. I remember the pleasure I had going into Barclay's Bank in Cockspur Street, which all South Africans in London seemed to patronize, to use the flush toilet in the ladies' room.

Sometimes, instead of Harry meeting me in London, I traveled the twelve miles by tube to his hospital to have a hot bath. In fact, my obsession about bathing became ridiculous. I'd become friendly with a Canadian woman doctor at the Hammersmith Institute who invited me to spend an evening with several friends at her fiancé's apartment in St. John's Wood. Water was expected to flow through the pipes in Dollis Hill that day, so I refused. My friend persisted and offered an inducement impossible to resist. She promised me a bath in her fiancé's apartment. I hesitated—longing to accept the offer, but feeling it was too much an imposition. With true camaraderie she agreed to ask her fiancé on my behalf, and I accepted happily. But when I arrived at the apartment, ahead of the other guests, and met her at the door, she hadn't yet broached the subject. Embarrassed though I was, my need overcame my hesitation. I told him my predicament and his fiancé's promise of a bath. Rather startled, but kind, he got up to get me towels. I thanked him warmly. "No need. I have everything with me," I said and produced my little suitcase. I wallowed in that bath in his lovely heated bathroom, my towels warm against the pipes. Never before or since have I felt such sensuous pleasure in bathing as I did then, luxuriating in that hot water and oblivious to the company outside. When I finally emerged, in a delicious torpor, I was in no mood for energetic conversation and left as soon as politeness allowed.

Neither the bathrooms nor the bedrooms where I became a

house officer (resident) were luxurious. House staff of the Queen's Hospital for Children slept in the attic, former servants' quarters, in rooms so small they held only a narrow iron bed, chest, and tiny closet. (I sympathized with the plight of the former inhabitants and imagined them running up and down stairs responding to bells.) On the other hand the English breakfasts were hearty, large, and good. (It's hard to spoil a breakfast.) We ate these breakfasts in the big dining room, helping ourselves to the hot porridge, boiling eggs to the consistency we preferred, and toasting the bread. Food was plentiful, and breakfast was leisurely. There was more staff for less work than I'd been accustomed to. To me British pace in all respects seemed more leisurely.

House staff impressed me enormously with their confidence that Britain could *not* be defeated, though daily they moved back the pins in the big wall map which showed Germany overrunning Europe. I'm certain that British belief in their own invincibility was a big factor in their final victory. My colleagues took me to nearby pubs and to the Prospect of Whitby, a pub well known in Dickens's time. They tried to get me to sample such delicacies as pickled eels, which I avoided, and taught me to play darts which I enjoyed. Only once did I impress them, when I diagnosed a young child as having congenital syphilis because of the shape of his teeth. Syphilis, uncommon in Britain, was so common in our South African patients that we automatically included it in our differential diagnosis of an illness.

Old and famous, the Queen's Hospital was located on Hackney Road in a poor section of London. The wards were only half full—all children well enough to be evacuated to the countryside had been sent there, and empty beds were earmarked for war casualties. I spent most of my time in the out-patient clinics and whenever possible listened to Dr. Helen McKay, renowned for her early research in rickets. I marveled at her patience, her modesty, her understanding of the mothers—all poor, many immigrants—and watched her repeated, careful demonstrations of the correct way to make up the baby's formula from dried milk powder and water, using readily available household measures and utensils. Another pediatrician, Dr. V. Mary Crosse, was equally impressive in her handling of premature babies and their mothers. Much later, when I came across the term "appropriate technology" usually used in connection with medical care in Third World countries, I remembered these doctors with their gas rings, kettles, cups, and teaspoons.

The day's work started later and ended earlier than in my South African job. In Port Elizabeth I had only alternate Sundays off duty; in London I had every other weekend off and some evenings. Whenever possible, Harry and I met in the West End during the week, and (against the rules) I spent my weekends off at his hospital.

The maid never really believed we were married. I remember the first time she found me in Harry's bedroom he was in the hospital doing a ward round. She stared at me, her eyes suspicious, while I nervously smoothed my hair with my left hand to show off my wedding ring, and told her who I was. After a moment of awkward silence, she pursed her thin lips, gave a loud sniff signifying disapproval of my loose foreign morals, and abruptly left the room. "Oh dear," I murmured, and then forgot about her for the next forty-five years.

Going our separate ways at night after meeting for a few hours was always wrenching. Returning to my hospital late at night in the blackout depressed me further. Afraid of being carried past the hospital and into Limehouse, I would sit near the driver and keep on reminding him to tell me when we neared my stop. Tourist London was unknown to me till years later—so many statues were sandbagged or removed for safety and heavy black curtains covered all doorways and windows.

One evening we decided to try a Hungarian restaurant in Soho for dinner. From the outside there was no way to distinguish expensive from cheaper places, but once we went through the curtained door the poshness of the place warned us that the prices would be beyond our limited means. The waiter brought a dish of pickled cucumbers to the table with our menus. The sight and smell of that delicious ethnic food—after months of bland, overcooked British fare—made our mouths water with desire. I remembered the sensation of eating a pickle taken straight out of my grandmother's wooden barrel, and I stretched out my hand to the dish on our table. Halfway there I restrained myself and looked at the menu prices. Harry and I whispered to each other planning our escape. Timorously I told the waiter that we were not hungry and "Could we just have salads?" Consulting with the manager, he reported back that we could not. Again I tried "Could we have soup alone?" Again the consultation and the same negative response. We told the waiter we were surprised that his restaurant was so inflexible, and in these circumstances we would have to leave. We rose, heads high, with no backward look at those tempting pickles, and left the restaurant with stern looks on our faces. Once outside the door we laughed till the tears came and could hardly wait till our next meeting with our close friends to repeat our tale.

We ate with Philip, Ben, and Basil whenever possible, usually at Lyons (eighteen pence for lunch and three pence extra for seconds of dessert) and Bertorellis for dinner (at least three courses for half a crown). For all of us eating provided a place to be together; food was less important than our happy companionship.

Philip, short and chubby, round-faced with a high forehead, a lovable butterball, with glasses perched on a small nose, was constantly in motion—talking, punning, gesticulating, laughing. Usually he wore a turtleneck sweater to save the costs of laundering shirts. Having lost his mother in his infancy, he had been brought up by an impoverished father and devoted older sisters and had earned his college tuition through tutoring schoolchildren. He was doing a Master's degree in English literature at the University of London and subsisting on a very small scholarship. Walking with Philip was a series of runs and stops, for he couldn't pass a display of secondhand books. Ben, not quite as hard pressed as Philip, but also on scholarship, was studying law in Gray's Inn. Tall and heavyset, his movements slow and deliberate, Ben spoke with a thick, small town, Cape accent. He told us of his childhood spent in a predominantly Afrikaner village where few Jewish families lived and of his father who had seven sons and who ruled over the Jewish community. Without the Beinart family it was impossible to have a *minyan*, the quorum of ten men required for religious services. If anyone disagreed with the patriarch, he would rise majestically, gather his sons together, and issue his command: "Come children!" That always ended the argument. Ben's father and Harry's father knew each other through some minor business dealings. One day, grinning broadly, Ben told us of a recent letter from his father expressing surprise at his friendship with the son of Phillips the *apikoros* (unbeliever). Besides English and Afrikaans, both Ben and Philip spoke fluent Hebrew as well as French, German, and Italian. Philip had more than a passing acquaintance with Latin and Greek; to Ben, Latin was still a living language.

A brilliant student, Basil at nineteen had been accepted for postgraduate study at the London School of Economics (LSE), having completed his undergraduate degree in economics at the University of Cape Town. Short, trim, always neatly turned out, with small features, high color and a ready smile, Basil was the youngest of us all.

Remembering those hours we spent together, listening to their sparkling conversation, their gaiety, wit, and humor, I think how lucky we were that our closest friends were not doctors. For they gave us an exciting introduction to fields other than our own. And in our serious times together they helped us to see South Africa in world perspective. It was Philip who later wrote that the world of imagination can't be carved up into "group areas."

But we couldn't for too long continue to focus on our personal careers. As South Africans, and as Jews, we wanted to help defeat Hitler. My father's oldest brother and his wife were victims of the Nazis in Warsaw; Harry's family also lost several relatives. So, it was time to return home when Italy entered the war, even though there was no conscription in South Africa. There would be fighting on the African continent, and Harry wanted to volunteer for service in the South African Medical Corps rather than in the British. In South Africa I could be near him, or near my family if he was posted overseas.

Before we left, I remembered my promise to my grandmother that I would be married in a synagogue. Someone directed us to a synagogue in St. John's Wood, and we arranged the details with the very pleasant rabbi. Ben insisted that he would be the one to give me away, and I walked down the aisle on his arm; the rabbi made a warm and rather touching speech; this time Philip was on time; Basil was there, and I had invited a young woman doctor from my hospital whom I liked very much and who wanted to see a Jewish wedding. There was also a very distant relative: Harry's brother-in-law, who'd grown up in Ireland and later emigrated to South Africa, had a sister in Leeds who decided she wanted to meet us and came to the wedding. Whether she felt sorry for me because I had no parents at the ceremony I don't know, but she acted like a mother who was sad to lose her daughter and wept under the marriage canopy. It really was a much nicer wedding than the one in the Marylebone town hall. Again we had a wonderful wedding lunch and then said farewells to our friends who would be staying on to complete their studies. They urged us to have a third wedding when we all met up again.

We have returned to London several times, for short visits and also for an extended period on sabbatical in 1980. After attending a lecture at the London School of Hygiene and Tropical Medicine, on our most recent visit, we walked along Gower Street going toward Tottenham Court Road to get back to our flat. Suddenly I realized we were in Charlotte Street and passing Bertorellis. Romantic that I am, I persuaded Harry that we should eat there, and I told the rather uninterested waiter and cashier how we had been good customers so many years ago. The prices were steep, the food not nearly as good as we remembered, but these are risks the sentimental must endure. We spoke of meals shared with our friends—two had died—and recalled the Yiddish proverb: Better one old friend than two new. Holding hands and remembering, we walked slowly to our flat.

Umtata: Rural Poverty

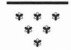

On our return from England Harry had gone to see the local deputy director of the South African Medical Corps to volunteer for military duty. He was told his services weren't required at that time, and he would be notified when he was needed. So we went for a seven-month internship to Umtata, the capital of the Transkei. For us it was a third short-term hospital internship, but the first in which we were both employed in the same hospital. Our dual appointment at the Sir Henry Elliot Hospital was most unusual—their first appointment of a married couple. I'd like to report that the hospital director disregarded custom because we were a particularly distinguished or desirable couple, but in truth the appointment was made reluctantly and purely for the convenience of the hospital. A new building for the medical staff wasn't finished; only two bedrooms were ready for three prospective house officers, and we two could share a room!

Coming directly from a year spent in London, we found the contrast between that city and Umtata immense. We left a densely crowded, sooty, blacked-out city, its statues sandbagged for protection, its radios and newspapers filled with war news, its children evacuated to the countryside, its pubs filled with proud people believing implicitly in their invincibility, accepting rationing and air-raid shelters with calmness and good humor. We arrived, in bright sunshine, at a small country town, part Western, part African. Umtata, the administrative center of a rural African Reserve was far into the interior and remote from war and thoughts of war. The Transkei, part of the Cape Province, was a relatively small area of about 16,000 square miles bounded by the Great Kei River in the south, the Indian Ocean in the east, Natal in the north, and Lesotho (formerly Basutoland) in the northwest. Its people subsisted mostly on corn, harvested by primitive methods and grown in red clay soil eroded, infertile, and overgrazed by cattle. These herds represented an integral part of the culture, signifying wealth, ancestral worship, *lobola*,[1] and food, mainly consumed as milk, for rarely were cattle slaughtered. Because the land had been depleted and its acreage become too small to support subsistence agriculture, the tax situation plus the activity of recruiting agents hastened the change to a new way of life. Able-bodied males became migrant laborers contracting for work on the mines, white farms, and in industry, returning to their rural homes for only a month or two each year. Many of these men also acquired "town wives" and families and a preference for urban life. As a consequence the Transkei that we saw had become the abode of old men, sick men, visiting men, and women and children.

The Transkei—and its health problems—was the product of the government's policy of restricting the black man's ownership of land. After the four provinces joined together to form the Union of South Africa, the government of Boers and Britons passed the Native Land Act of 1913 which established segregation in land ownership and occupation.[2] Through this notorious Act most of the land formerly occupied by Africans was given to whites, and Africans—who at that time already made up more than two-thirds of the estimated total population of South Africa—were squeezed into 12 percent of the land.

These black areas, over time, were called Scheduled Areas, Native Territories, Native Reserves, Bantustans, Homelands, and finally Independent States. Similarly, the names given to the Africans by the white man changed from Kaffirs (from the Arabic meaning heathens), to Natives, Bantu (an ethnic and linguistic classification), Africans, and more recently (following American usage) Blacks. All male residents of these Scheduled Areas, at age eighteen, were subjected to a Poll Tax, which had to be paid in cash. The pressures of too little land plus the need for tax money were powerful weapons to ensure a plentiful supply of black labor for white enterprises.

The largest of these reserves were the Transkeian territories in the Cape Province and Zululand in Natal. As doctors we worked with the people of both these areas—at least with their health problems—most of which, as I've said, stemmed directly from the government's policy of forced separation of the races—known later as apartheid. It is a sad reflection on government policy that I can give no accurate figures on the extent of illness and death in these black communities. The reason is simple; these statistics do not, even now, exist.

In South Africa, except for some notifiable infectious diseases, there are no regularly published national, provincial, or local sickness reports for all its people. Data on deaths are collected, but even here there are limitations with regard to blacks. While the numbers of deaths by cause, age, and sex are published for whites, Asians, and coloreds in the whole country, deaths for blacks have been reported only in recent years and even then only for the main urban areas. Census figures for blacks are known only for those who live in white urban areas. Even infant mortality rates are not universally available for blacks. The information we have on the deaths of black babies comes from medical officers of health in a few major cities and can only be regarded as estimates.[3]

As I recall, Umtata had an undistinguished main street sloping downhill, and several country stores catering to the few whites and the many blacks of the town and surrounding areas. Near the center of the town, in one of the few imposing buildings, the Paramount Chief met with his tribal advisory council: the Bunga. Houses of the white population were clustered around the main street, but the Africans of the town lived in the segregated location in housing provided by the municipality.

One of my many duties was to attend a weekly well-baby clinic in this location about two miles from the hospital, reached by a narrow dirt road full of potholes. I quickly learned where these holes were because when they filled up with rain it wasn't easy or safe to drive without such knowledge.

High on a plateau on the edge of town stood the hospital with an unobstructed view of the distant hills and mountains. It had 211 beds and served the million people of the Transkei. Another forty beds housed the white patients of the local practitioners. It wasn't the only hospital in the Transkei, but the others were much smaller and mostly run by Protestant medical missionaries. All severe cases and emergencies came to the hospital in Umtata.

There were a few smaller towns in the Transkei, but most Africans were rural and lived in clusters of traditional housing—small one-room huts made of wattle and daub, with hard dung floors and thatched roofs. Cooking was done in big iron pots over open fires. The staple foods were corn (eaten as thick porridge), beans, pumpkins, wild greens, and soured milk. Beer was both a food and a drink, made by the women from a type of sorghum (called red Kaffir corn). Beer played an essential role in the life of the community, freely given in hospitality at all festive and ceremonial occasions. Along with sacrifices of fowls or goats, beer was offered to the ancestors at important times such as birth, marriage, or sickness, and to propitiate them for any inadvertent breach of custom.

The soil's red color was repeated in the ocher blankets worn by the pipe-smoking Xhosas. The women, bare to the waist, were often elaborately beaded and wondrously coiffed. There were different traditional styles of dress for maidens and matrons as well as different hair styles. In one style married women displayed twisted, ochered braids of hair piled high on the head with an elaborate filling of red clay and fat. The hairdo might last as much as six months, and women wore implements, shaped somewhat like knitting needles, stuck through the headdress for decoration and used also to scratch when necessary. The women were comely. They walked erect with the grace of dancers, babies firmly ensconced on their backs in a shawled nest, loads of firewood or buckets of water balanced on their heads.

Men walked free of burdens, although at times a precious pair of shoes, tied together by their laces, dangled from a neck. When a man rode on horseback, his wife followed on foot, but never did I see that pattern reversed.

We learned that a woman's main duty was bearing children, though she also worked hard in other ways. She fetched water (often from long distances), collected firewood, prepared mud bricks, cleaned house, stamped grain, made beer, cooked food, cultivated fields, and fashioned baskets, sleeping mats, and clay pots for holding water and beer. Men's traditional duties were fighting, herding and milking, hunting, sitting in judgment, and deciding on policy. With the introduction of the plough (drawn by oxen) men also tilled the fields, since women were prohibited by religious sanction from contact with cattle. However, when the men were away from home working in the cities, women, willy-nilly, had to plough. From an early age children were given duties, again determined by their sex. Little girls helped their mothers with all domestic duties and acted as nursemaids for their younger siblings. It was common to see a small girl carrying a still smaller one on her back. Little boys herded—first the kids, later the goats and calves, and finally full cattle herds.

Between Harry and me the only gender-related difference, with regard to our hospital duties, was that he was automatically regarded as senior to me. Even though, for reasons I don't recall, I began the job a month before he did, from the moment he arrived he was the one to be turned to if we were together. We worked long hours with no let up, beginning with ward rounds at eight each morning and continuing till six in the evening. Night duty began at six, and even if we'd been up all night we were expected to carry on as usual the following day. With a full complement of three medical house staff, we were each on night duty one night in three; this meant literally being up all night. But one night in three each of us was also second on call and usually it was necessary at least once to get up and assist. One night in three, each had a full night's sleep. The one disadvantage in sharing a bedroom was the telephone. Harry woke when he was the first on call, but not when I was; I, a light sleeper, woke whenever the phone rang. Most of the time there were three house officers, but for one incredible six-week period there were just the two of us to do all the work. The director of the hospital took pity on us one night and took over our calls for the evening hours. He sent us to the movies where we slept through the entire show, blissfully undisturbed.

Three local doctors in private practice acted as "honoraries" to the hospital and supervised our work. Two were general practitioners, one of whom did all the major surgery. He had an assistant, a young doctor previously employed at the hospital. The third and oldest practitioner, a gentle person, was reputed to be struggling against a longtime morphine addiction. He seemed to develop a cough whenever he came to the hospital and asked the nursing staff for a dose of linctus heroin, commonly used at that time to suppress a dry, irritating cough. The director of the hospital, a doctor himself, did no clinical work. After we'd been at work for two or three months, the director encouraged us to set up an ambulatory clinic at the hospital—a new service for patients. Until that time (apart from emergencies) almost all patients we saw were referred for direct in-patient admission by the practitioners of the town or from doctors in other towns or mission hospitals. Provincial hospital services were free for Africans, but physicians in private practice charged fees when patients saw them in their offices, plus an additional small fee for operative procedures in the hospital. Not surprisingly, the doctors considered the hospital's ambulatory clinic to be an infringement on their private practice and voiced their displeasure.

We ourselves were paid the usual medical house staff pittance of the day, plus board and lodging, and never questioned the meager salaries of the time. In fact we thought very little about the whole question of how health services were financed—the subject had never been mentioned in the six years of our medical training. Doctors didn't consider this to be an issue for their concern—it was a matter for administrators to handle.

Considering the paucity of doctors and the large numbers of people needing medical care, it was understandable that we carried out procedures every day that in a big city would only be done by persons far senior to ourselves. Antibiotics were not yet in general use, nor was there a blood transfusion service in place. The hospital had an X-ray machine and a small laboratory, but no radiologist, pathologist, or technicians to service them. Each departing house officer taught the incoming doctor to handle the medical and technical tasks. I shudder now to think how blithely we used fluoroscopy to visualize chests or to remove foreign bodies. We and our patients must have been exposed to grossly unsafe levels of radiation whose effects would be with us the rest of our lives.

There were medical and surgical wards for men and women, infectious disease wards (tuberculosis was rampant), an obstetric ward, and two children's wards divided by age rather than sex. Though I did a great deal of minor surgery, I was never in charge of surgical wards. At different times I looked after all the other divisions and, happily, cared for the children's wards for the full seven months of my stay—acquiring the African name of "the doctor who loves babies."

We marveled at the physical stamina, endurance, and courage of the people. The hospital's two ambulances picked up people up to a radius of forty miles, but patients had to make their own way to pickup points, often from faraway. Requests for ambulance service were frequently relayed by the owners of rural trading stations. We, in turn, might send a message to a trader that a patient was due for discharge and would be dropped off at a particular trading store. Once when I became very impatient at the inordinate delay of an ambulance, I protested to the driver of the second ambulance. "What can you expect from a Pondo?" he replied. To my natural follow-up question, "And what are you?" he answered shamefacedly, "I'm a Pondo, Doctor." Is there *any* society without hierarchical prejudice?

Many times men arrived on horseback, and if there were two together we mightn't know which one needed care until their blankets were removed, exposing the wounds on the injured one. On one occasion, two men rode in. One had been hit on the head with a *knobkerrie* (a club); his friend, exploring the wound with a feather to see how deep it went, reported that he'd seen something like marrow on the feather! Amazingly sepsis didn't occur and ten days later the patient rode back home.

A young man walked in one day with a fractured humerus. He'd broken his arm six years earlier and had developed a false joint; we never got a proper explanation of why he'd waited so long to come for treatment. On the other hand, a mother walked one hundred miles in three or four days with her baby on her back when she noticed the baby had developed a scrotal swelling. She'd heard that I was good with babies and fortunately the condition was easily rectified.

People came suffering from typhoid fever, pneumonia, diphtheria, tuberculosis, syphilis in all its stages, malnutrition including kwashiorkor, scurvy and pellagra, worm infestations, schistosomiasis, and other parasitic infections. They survived trauma but had little resistance to tuberculosis.

We practiced heroic medicine, but we were ignorant of Xhosa history and culture, and our contacts were limited to the medical domain. We didn't yet know how the migrant labor system completely upset the stability of the family and the traditional male/female relationships. We had no real grasp of colonial history, usually written to the advantage of the colonial power, and we concentrated on our biological knowledge of illness. I'm certain we were not then conscious that the Xhosa subsistence agricultural economy was being rapidly replaced by a monetary system dependent on cash remittances from absent husbands. Gradually we began to learn that most of the men who came for treatment of venereal disease or were admitted to the hospital with advanced TB (and who had likely infected their families) had been laboring, usually in the mines, and were sent home when too sick to continue working.

Of one thing, however, we were acutely conscious: our inability to speak or understand the Xhosa language caused an almost

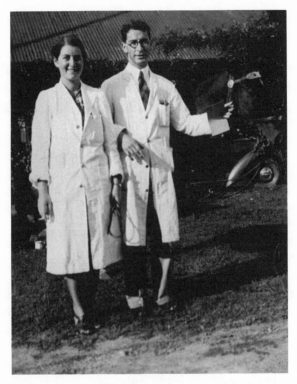

With patient's horse and, in those days, cigarettes

unbridgeable gap between us. While examining patients we could ask them, in Xhosa, to breathe deeply or to cough, and we even learned to ask a few simple questions. But what was the use when we couldn't understand their answers? Forced always to use interpreters, we often wondered what nuances we were missing. It was maddening when at times the simplest question such as "Does he have any pain?" might evoke a torrent of words to the interpreter, but to us only the monosyllabic "Yes" or "No." It was easier to communicate with small children, for body language told much. A smile, soothing murmurs, arms held out to pick up an infant, a touch, a pat, or a warm hug conveyed our caring emotions.

We liked the people very much and admired their dignified patience, their stoicism, their good humor, their love of children. But every day brought fresh problems: patients' horses had to be kept and fed until their owners recovered and could ride home again. And of course every mother wanted to stay with her baby. I allowed mothers of breast-fed babies under nine months of age to stay with them, and if mothers came from a great distance, I amended my own rules. Though I knew so little of the culture, even then I appreciated the oneness of the Xhosa mother-baby connection. Waiting with heads bowed, mothers never questioned my decisions—at least not in my presence. Fortunately, most were able to stay. They slept on the floor beside their babies' cots.

I learned many simple lessons as I went along. At that time pediatric wisdom dictated regular feedings every four hours. But Xhosa mothers nursed their babies for comfort as well as for food, and they had no clocks. So I gave up that idea in short order. I also stopped keeping children in bed when they felt better. When children felt ill they stayed in bed, but as soon as possible they climbed out of their cots and joined their playmates outdoors. Their behavior seemed perfectly sensible to me. During daylight hours the children's wards had very few occupants.

The empty wards posed great problems for Pikili—a courageous and stoic, shiny-skinned beautiful little boy of three to whom I lost my heart at first sight. He arrived by ambulance (his home village eighty miles away) with a fractured thigh bone, and I put his broken leg in a gallows splint, held in position by a counterweight. Pikili lay in bed on his back, his left leg extended in the air and immobilized by the splint. He was, so to speak, hung by the leg and couldn't get out of bed. Daily I watched him coaxing children to stay near him to play instead of going outdoors; his charm and sweet nature was such that he sometimes succeeded. He also managed to maneuver himself so well that I'd find him rolled over on his side when it suited his games, and I had to threaten suspension of both legs to prevent him from excessive movement of the broken leg.

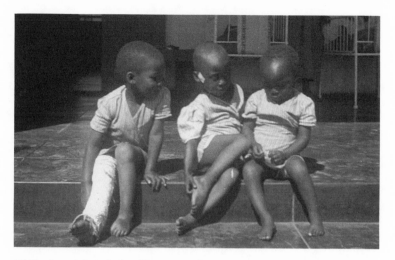

Pikili released from bed and soon to go home

In due course his bone healed, and I took off the splint. Pikili was free, but I was sad to lose him. Each day I put off his departure, telling the nurse he must be surefooted before we could reasonably let him go. Then one night as I approached the threshold of the ward to do my usual evening round, I saw Belinda, the oldest child in the ward (slowly recovering from severe burns), doing a ward round, pretending to be me. I recognized myself in my walk and gestures as she slowly went from bed to bed, smiling at one child, chatting to another, touching a third. Then she came to Pikili's bed, threw her arms around him, and hugged him. The message of my favoritism was all too clear. Guiltily, next morning I gave the orders for his discharge. But even now, so many years later, I see that little face and those big, brown eyes and wonder what has become of him. He may be a father, perhaps a grandfather by now, but for me, always a little boy who captured my heart.

I can take no personal credit for one remarkable cure. When I took over the children's ward, there was a little girl in a side room. She had *cancrum oris*, a condition which I'd come across only in textbooks and which I never again encountered. Resulting from a combination of severe malnutrition and very bad infection, this disease shows itself as a chronic ulcer of the cheek which erodes right through the tissues. There cannot have been many survivors in the preantibiotic days, but our nursing staff were determined that the child would recover, even though they had no specific therapy available to them. Tenderly, they fed and nursed the little girl, dressed the wound gently, and gave her unfailing attention. It seemed to me that she was bathed in love. When I left she was still in hospital, but about to be discharged.

I've mentioned earlier that young boys helped their fathers herd cattle. One of their tasks was to lead the ox-drawn wagons. Sometimes a front ox became irritable, lowered his head, and gored the young lad with his horns: a rural occupational disease. These ox-pokes produced wounds in the buttock area which invariably became septic. Happily all our patients recovered.

But this was not the case with newborn babies with tetanus. These babies became unable to suck when they developed lockjaw because their cheek muscles went into spasm, and as their condition worsened, these spasms spread over the entire body. It was an excruciatingly painful and almost always fatal disease for the little sufferer and terrible to witness, yet this disease was completely preventable. It usually happened because the "granny midwife," after cutting the umbilical cord, dressed it with cow dung—a grim lesson to us on the need for skilled birth care. Certainly, many of the difficult deliveries I was faced with could have been prevented by health education.

The nursing sister in charge of midwifery was well-trained, but because she was a nurse and I a doctor—though not nearly as experienced—she was allowed to deliver normal births only. Anything requiring forceps, or other intervention, had to be done by a doctor. I was a willing pupil and learned most of my practical midwifery from the Umtata nurses—we had no lack of births. There was a very special satisfaction in being able to present a lusty, healthy baby to its eagerly waiting mother.

I think it's worth noting that in the seven months of my stay, I never heard a single African mother groan aloud in labor!

The importance of singing to African people came as a revelation. The wards of men and women each had at least sixteen beds and were separated from each other by a wide corridor. At sundown they sang—one ward beginning the melody, the other harmonizing—their voices strong and clear in the still night air, their sorrows forgotten a while in the music they made. There seemed to be a feeling of togetherness, of community, in that chorus of voices. We listened entranced with its beauty. Not knowing the meaning of the words, we could appreciate fully only the loveliness of their harmonies. So strongly were we moved that to this day African singing has the same emotional effect on us—particularly when we hear *Nkosi Sikelel' i Afrika*— God Bless Africa, which invariably makes us cry.

Patients certainly knew about each other and what treatment we gave each one. Because screens, to patients, signified impending death we avoided their use as much as possible. One woman, malnourished, bedridden, semiparalyzed, and mentally confused, had been in the medical ward some time before I took it over. I treated her pellagra because I wanted to do something for her, but not because I thought it had anything to do with her overall condition, for I hadn't known that pellagra could affect the nervous system. To my surprise and great pleasure she improved greatly, becoming more rational and even beginning to walk again. I was so delighted with her recovery that I wrote a letter to the South African Medical Journal reporting her case. The women of the ward were as pleased as I was, and the news of her cure soon spread across the corridor to the men's ward.

Adult men sometimes proved more difficult to cope with. An old man with a gray beard came in for retention of urine due to an old gonorrheal urethral stricture. As was the custom for many men, he wore a prepuce cover. The treatment prescribed for him was to have his stricture gradually stretched and to insert a catheter to allow a flow of urine. He was not my patient, but since there were only three of us, all patients knew our night duty roster. I was awakened one night because the *kehle* (old man) had pulled out his catheter. I put it back without incident, and he gave no trouble until I was again on night duty. Again I was awakened to reinsert the catheter. Displeased as I was at being disturbed because of his deliberate action, I didn't, at first, notice his mischievous grin and the twinkle in his eye as I began to put back the catheter. But at the age of twenty-four, how the devil was I supposed to deal with a man old enough to be my grandfather, tickled pink that he was having an erection (which I was pretending not to notice) while I was holding onto a fast disappearing catheter!

We often used procedures in the men's medical ward simply to lighten illnesses for which we had no cure. There were always one or two men with cirrhosis of the liver and abdomens full of fluid, and to relieve the pressure we would tap the abdomen with a trocar, insert a tube, and drain the fluid into a container. Very commonly, too, there'd be men with urethral strictures whose urine would be draining through tubes. To us these procedures had become commonplace, but in one week when I'd already done an abdominal tap and relieved a stricture, a man was admitted with severe difficulty in breathing because of accumulation of fluid in his chest due to an infection of the lining surrounding the lung. Again I removed fluid—this time with a large needle and syringe.

The morning after this last procedure, I noticed a difference in the ward atmosphere when I did my usual rounds. There seemed to be a strange mixture of deference coupled with some uneasiness on the part of nurses as well as patients, rather than the usual friendliness with which I was customarily greeted. With some reluctance the nurses explained: I had drawn fluid from three different parts of the body. I had made a paralyzed woman walk. I had given proof of my calling. I was endowed with supernatural powers, not a witch doctor who does evil deeds, but certainly a magical healer! Quite firmly I denied my supposed magical powers, though there were many times

I wished I had them, and after a while we seemed to resume normal relationships.

So far I have written only about the people we served and the kind of work we did, for those matters occupied us to the full. As medical residents we had little time for relaxation—a movie, perhaps an excursion or two. We had one wonderful weekend at Coffee Bay on the magnificent Wild Coast of the Transkei. The third house officer, whom we had helped to do a six-week locum for a job he wanted, repaid us by taking over our duties for a weekend. Strangely, I remember nothing at all about the kind of food we ate, where it was served—presumably in a white, staff dining room—or other details of daily living. All I seem to remember are the patients. But we did go to one party.

On New Year's Eve we were invited to a party given by the matron (nursing director) and senior nursing staff. I wore my long evening dress, as was the fashion of the time, though I doubt that Harry wore a tuxedo. What I recall most vividly about that night was that after the toasts to the New Year had been drunk, we donned our obligatory paper hats, linked arms, and went from ward to ward doing a dual ward round before finally going to bed. We were to have a busy New Year's day.

In Cape Town we were accustomed to the New Year being celebrated with far more jollity than Christmas, but we didn't know whether Africans celebrated these holidays the same way. We discovered that because it was a public holiday, and therefore a day of leisure, there was increased drinking and subsequent fighting; as a result Harry spent most of the day stitching wounds, setting fractures, and even trephining a skull with a depressed fracture. I was just as busy. Among other emergencies I saw two mothers in obstructed labor. The cause of the obstruction was the same in each of the women—a distended bladder which by the time of admission could be relieved only by catheterization. Birth contractions had begun four days earlier in each mother, and their babies were already dead. I was lucky to save the mothers. I remember, clearly, how upset and frustrated I was at the unnecessary suffering of the mothers and the loss of their babies, and I remember asking the Xhosa nurses to send messages to the Paramount Chief. I wanted him to instruct all mothers nearing labor to empty their bladders at regular intervals. But I don't know if my messages were sent or, if sent, were heeded. New Year's Day, 1941—a day we won't likely forget.

Forty-two years passed before we returned to the Transkei. We went back to the Sir Henry Elliot Hospital in Umtata when we visited South Africa in the spring of 1983. The Transkei had graduated from a Bantustan to an "independent state," recognized as such only by George Matanzima, the prime minister, by his henchmen, and by the South African government. Foreigners needed a permit to enter the Transkei in addition to the South African visa, but when we were stopped at the barrier, the officials seemed only to be interested in our car license number and the names and numbers of our passengers. Nobody asked to see our permit. In this South African puppet state, the trappings of pseudo-authority were a cold and disturbing reminder of Pretoria's legislative designs, and I thought of Sir Thomas More's words, written almost five hundred years earlier, about the ways of the rich with the poor.

"Therefore when I consider and weigh in my mind all these commonwealths . . . I can perceive nothing but a certain conspiracy of rich men, procuring their own commodities under the name and title of the commonwealth. They invent and devise all means and crafts first how to keep safely . . . that they have unjustly gathered together; and next how to hire and abuse the work and labor of the poor. . . . These devices, when the rich men have decreed to be kept and observed for the commonwealth's sake . . . then they be made laws." [4]

In the morning we saw something of Umtata. The municipal office had no maps to give us, but staff kindly copied some from a book they had. We spoke of the weather and the devastating drought and were told if the rains didn't come by September all the cattle would be dead. They asked us to pray for rain. A South African military truck passed by, distributing water to the most distressed rural areas. As we drove in we saw the uniformly brown and red earth, with no trace of green, a few sheep, but no sign of cattle. The park in the center of town, enclosing the city hall, was still watered and cared for, providing some color.

Numerous Africans sat on the wall of the new Bunga across from the park and went in and out of the buildings in a constant stream. The town had grown significantly; the center seemed moderately prosperous. We asked the officials about the presence of a museum. There was one, immediately across from the office we had gone to, but they didn't know what was in it. Our hearts were no longer in the visit, and we didn't explore. But we asked for directions to the Sir Henry Elliot Hospital.

The hospital now serviced only TB patients. A new general hospital, which we didn't visit, had been built, but the old hospital seemed completely unchanged. The basic structure of single-story separate buildings, each with its long, roofed verandah running alongside, seemed just as we had left it—perhaps a little shabbier. We introduced ourselves to the nurses, and I asked to see the children's ward. As usual there were more children outside the ward than in it. The nurses assembled the children, sat them down on the steps leading from the long porch to the flat grounds, and told them to sing for us. Once more we loved the sound of the songs, and once again we did not know the meanings of the words.

Cape Town: 1941

On two occasions, widely separated in time, Harry and I worked in Cape Town: after returning from Umtata in 1941 and again in 1954 after leaving the Institute of Family and Community Health in Durban. In 1941 we had no children; by 1954 we had four. No other city evoked in us the same joy of place as did Cape Town with its extraordinary beauty, its sense of history, its familiarity. Both times we knew our stay would be temporary—the 1941 return would end when Harry was called up for military service, the 1954 stay when a job in another country would enable us to emigrate. But we fitted into the rhythm of the city we were born in easily and gladly.

We rented an apartment on our first time back—it was our first real home together—furnished it scantily but lovingly,and lived in it for less than a year. Still waiting for his military call (it took more than a year between his volunteering and his induction), Harry got a job as assistant to a firm of doctors whose major practice consisted of contracts with shipowners to treat their merchant marine ships' crews during docking in Cape Town harbor. As a result of World War II the Suez Canal and the Mediterranean were closed to British and Allied craft, and ships traveled the long route to the East via the Cape. At times Cape Town harbor was swollen with vessels. After Harry saw the sick sailors, he left a bill with the ship's captain detailing the charges. It wasn't long before he realized that he earned for his firm in one day what they paid him for a month's work! But his work was interesting and enlightening, as was his vocabulary, enriched by mixing with the American sailors. Most importantly

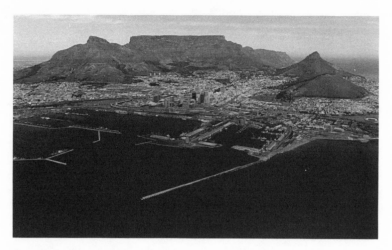

Cape Town from the air

his tenure was flexible; he could be released immediately when called to service.

Every evening Harry would tell me of that day's adventures. When the docks were choked with ships, several would be tightly berthed side by side making access to the farthest ship possible only by climbing the ladder of the nearest one, followed by clambering from boat to boat to reach the last one. Out in the bay climbing the boarding ladder was no mean task, needing nimble footwork and timing with the swell of the water.

Early, Harry recognized the chronic emotional stress from which wartime sailors suffered and the effects of this stress on their health. Men were at sea for long stretches of time; for those whose countries had been overrun early, like Norway and Holland, return to home port and families wasn't possible, adding gloom and anxiety to the sometimes appalling physical conditions on board. Blackout precautions added to physical discomfort. Many British ships used Lascar (Indian) seamen, housed them poorly, fed them badly, and treated them with very little consideration. Officers and men were literally and figuratively from different worlds.

By far the best ships were American. Harry was impressed by the difference in cleanliness and comfort, by the lack of deference and subservience shown by the men toward their superior officers, and by the ribald language used so freely in their altercations. The trade union movement had done much for the seamen, and they were very conscious of their rights. When Harry needed to climb a ship's ladder, a line would be thrown to him for attachment to his bag of instruments in order to haul it aboard. On one occasion he asked an idle American sailor leaning over the rail for a line. "Sorry Doc," came the laconic reply, "I'm off duty. What time is it?" Told it was a quarter of three the sailor grinned. "Don't come on till three, Doc; I'll ask my mate to help you." But aside from the Americans (who had not yet come into the war) a large number of sailors led a miserable life under these wartime conditions.

German submarines lurked at Cape Agulhas, the southernmost tip of Africa, ready to attack British and Allied ships whose movements were reported to Germany by pro-Nazi sympathizers. As a result, numerous ships were torpedoed before they reached the safety of Cape Town harbor or after they left. Harry's patients included some men who were badly burned or suffering from exposure before they could be rescued from lifeboats or from the sea itself. On the way down the west coast of Africa, convoys of ships put in at Free Town in Sierra Leone where many sailors contracted venereal diseases. One particularly dangerous disease was malaria—endemic in Sierra Leone. By the time those who were infected reached Cape Town, they were usually very sick. When ships could not dock, doctors went out to them by launch; once Harry went by tugboat to bring in a man desperately ill with cerebral malaria. He still talks with wonderment of this comatose, seemingly dying man, dramatically restored to life by large injections of quinine.

On merchant ships the first officer acted as medic, screening patients and giving first aid. His standard manual was filled with simple, often humorous, nautical language; for example, it informed the reader that appendicitis manifested itself by pain which settled in the southwest corner of the abdomen! Patients in need of hospitalization were brought to a private hospital in Sea Point called the Monastery, staffed by Catholic nuns who were excellent nurses giving dedicated care. Friendly women, they were acquainted with the partners of the medical firm which Harry assisted. Every year a wealthy Catholic businessman lent the nuns his large seaside house, with its private swimming pool, as a holiday retreat. Once we happened to be spending a weekend at this small resort village, during one of these holiday periods, and the nuns invited us to tea. We came upon them frolicking in the pool, unabashedly having a lot of noisy fun, swimming in their modest bathing suits with unveiled heads revealing their very close cropped hair. At tea they behaved like a bunch of jolly, giggling, almost flirtatious, schoolgirls, a side we did not see when, clothed in their ample habits, they carried out their serious work at the hospital.

A small part of Harry's work, apart from his shipping duties, included helping in the doctors' private practice at their office and in their clients' homes—caring for their poorest and most troublesome patients. Here he learned another side of life. One of the doctors' regular patients assigned to him soon after he joined the firm (for reasons which became obvious later) was a neurotic middle-aged woman whose many complaints always needed a thorough physical examination. Never finding any organic reason for her symptoms, but being called very frequently, Harry became suspicious of her motives and increasingly worried that she was trying to seduce him. One night she called our apartment late insisting that she was very ill, that he must come immediately to see her at home, that she could *not* wait until the following morning. Unaccustomed to dealing with this type of patient and reluctant to go alone, Harry turned to me for support. We visited her together. While I was being introduced, I noticed that she was wearing a "see-through" nightgown. Although I waited in another room while Harry examined her, after this visit she didn't ask for him to see her again and went back to calling for the senior partners.

Just as the impact of actually going onto the ships and seeing the environment in which the seamen lived left an indelible impression on Harry, so these house calls were necessary for our shared education. One longtime client of the firm was a poor, immigrant Jewish shoemaker with a large family. A home visit to confirm the diagnosis of measles in a young son, during which Harry gave reassurance but no prescription, resulted in a phone call the next day to a senior partner to say how nice the young doctor had been, but they would like the older doctor to come as well since they had gotten no medicine for the child. Harry went back to this family several times, always after that prescribing some potion, but he hated writing out a bill for them. An experience like this was one of the reasons which steered Harry away from private practice and into public health.

Since the timing of Harry's military call-up was so uncertain, I was left with few options for jobs. Private practice had absolutely no appeal for me. My dislike of (what I have now learned to call) a fee-for-service type of system, a mixing of medicine with money, was intensified by Harry's experience and by my work with the poverty-stricken Africans of Port Elizabeth and Umtata. But neither could I get involved in any salaried job that would mean a lasting commitment. As a temporary measure I accepted a six months job, which could be extended to twelve months, at the Cape Town Free Dispensary, a municipal, free-standing, ambulatory clinic serving a mainly colored, but also a poor white clientele. The clinic, which had long been known by its less educated clients as the Cape Town "Free Expenses," was very popular, and a large proportion of the colored people in central Cape Town regarded it as their family doctor.

In many ways this job was similar to my first one in Port Elizabeth, but it had several advantages. For me the greatest benefit was that I had joined another doctor, a young woman senior to me who had graduated from medical school a year before I did. The needs of the people I saw were again largely social, economic, and environmental, hardly to be touched by our limited, palliative medical care, but it was far less stressful when bracing myself against the daily onslaught to know that I did not have to face this alone.

Mary came from a wealthy and far more sophisticated background than mine; she was bright, extremely attractive, and fun to be with. She entertained me with stories, during lunch breaks, about her numerous boyfriends none of whom knew of each other's existence. Though Mary and I managed to treat most of our patients without outside help, there were some consultant sessions attended by very senior doctors to whom we referred patients. The most dramatic sessions of all were conducted by an ear-nose-and-throat surgeon who later became the first Minister of Health when the Nationalist Party came into power. Tuesday mornings were notable for the number of children who came to part with their tonsils and adenoids.[1] Taking turns, Mary and I were always present at the specialist sessions; at times we were ordered to take out a few tonsils for practice. The method then in vogue was quick and bloody. Our surgeon often missed the pail specially provided for dumping the guillotined tonsils; the floor around us was slippery with blood. On days without attending specialists, we could if necessary refer patients to the emergency room, or the clinics, of the Groote Schuur Hospital. But we two young doctors were expected to handle, at least to screen, most of the problems ourselves—sore throats, coughs, pneumonia, gastroenteritis, scabies, impetigo, tuberculosis, venereal diseases, alcoholism, trauma, etc.

Another gain over the Port Elizabeth job was my knowledge of Afrikaans, the mother tongue of the Afrikaners and of the colored people. And the culture of this population was more familiar—akin as it was to that of the whites. At the Free Dispensary we could talk together and understand each other, however brief the interaction.

There were other reasons, also, why I was better able to cope. By this time I had grown some of the protective shell doctors need to function in a situation where medical care can do little to ease the problems their patients face. I noticed, too, with passing interest, that I had become dulled to gender; it had become as natural for me to examine a man as a woman. Without a second thought I would tell men with a history of gonorrhea to "please go into that cubicle and pull your pants down so I can examine you." Patients had little choice since both staff doctors happened to be women.

Of course by this time I could manage better because my skills had increased. I was much more experienced and confident—to the point of reluctantly agreeing to Harry's demand that I be the one to remove a sebaceous cyst behind his left ear. (I looked for the scar when I was writing this sentence, but could no longer find it. We both laughed aloud remembering how Harry had teased me throughout the procedure telling me I was cutting into his brain while I tried to be firm and get him to keep his head, and his tongue, still!)

Harry was called up after I had been at the Dispensary for ten months, first to training camp—known colloquially as the chain gang—and then to a base hospital in Ladysmith, Natal. I was asked to stay on my job an extra month or two until I could be replaced, after which I joined him.

In retrospect two things stand out most clearly from my Dispensary experience: the one emotional, the other practical. However frustrating the job, I had enjoyed working with the people. My warm attitude toward colored people had developed early because of my deep childhood attachment to Sakkie. I felt that Cape Town's colored people had a directness in their acceptance of life and a capacity for enjoyment, in spite of their hardships, that we inhibited whites, with our privileges, fears, and guilt feelings, lacked. But there was another and painful side to their acceptance of their lot which they—like Jews—expressed in their joking, inwardly turned humor, the bitter laughter of those whom Sarah Gertrude Millin called God's stepchildren.

Yet despite, or perhaps because of, my liking for colored people, after that year of work I vowed never to take such a job again. I knew by then what I wanted in my future: to go back to school and get a public health degree, to tackle the root causes of ill health and try to prevent them, to work in a setting where I had time to know my patients and they me, to work with others who felt the same way that Harry and I did.

A short while back, in Chapel Hill, North Carolina, we watched a company of black South African male performers who called themselves Ladysmith Black Mambazo and, after a gap of over forty years, half-forgotten memories of my life as a war wife in Ladysmith surfaced.

The most joyous of these recollections were of David who was born during that time—though not in Ladysmith. As a new mother I was taking no second best for my baby and went to Cape Town for the delivery. I've had few pleasures greater than witnessing my babies' growth and development and the miracle of speech entrances me. David's first real word at ten months was "flower," though only a proud parent might have recognized it. My saddest memory was seeing the pain of another war wife who visited weekly to use my baby scale and who refused for the longest time to acknowledge that her son was retarded.

But apart from my immediate family, for me that year was a try- ing period of suspension—an unmoored, floating waiting until the war would end and we could again choose our town, our friends, our work. Military hospital staff formed a closed society—hardly mixing with the white, civilian population of the town, let alone its Indian and black residents. An air of almost feverish gaiety prevailed, with parties, drinking, short-lived affairs—a grabbing of pleasure before facing possible death. Having no job I eased my conscience somewhat by part-time volunteer service in the baby clinics of the segregated, black township, but a gap remained.

Some months after David's birth, I moved from my Ladysmith hotel room to a rented house on the outskirts of the town, which I shared with another army wife. Our husbands lived in hospital quarters but had fairly liberal off-duty hours. The very first night in that lodging showed us the disadvantage of living next to

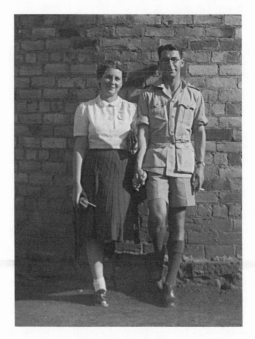

With my army husband on leave

uncultivated fields. The house was infested with huge rats that ate *everything* not enclosed. When I found rat-droppings on the mosquito netting covering David's crib, with him in my arms, I marched to the health department and demanded the services of a ratcatcher. The department had no such person and owned but six rattraps which they baited with cheese—toasted, they told me, to enhance the flavor. Each evening they set the traps; each morning they removed six dead rats. But after a week of this activity, they decided I could no longer have their entire ratcatching resources. I was on my own. Luckily, our housemates were only waiting to get settled before reclaiming their two terriers from boarding kennels in Johannesburg. While the dogs sometimes shared David's toys and bones, our rat problems were over.

Every South African who volunteered for foreign war service—there was no conscription—wanted to get to Italy. Fortunately for me Harry didn't get further than Egypt. My housemate, Stella, a good cook, had taught me the simplest cookie recipe she knew, and I had just put a batch in the oven when Harry came to tell me he'd gotten his marching orders for "up North." Only the smell of burning reminded me I'd been baking, and I've had an aversion to making cookies ever since.

David and I returned to live in my parents' home, and I went back to school to study public health. Eighteen months later, when Harry was finally repatriated, and I knew the time his train from Pretoria would arrive in Cape Town station, I planned to surprise him. I took a local train to Worcester, a stopping point about two hours up the road, and hopped onto his train hoping he hadn't seen me waiting on the platform. But I'd forgotten the length of those trains and, as I peered through the glass of innumerable compartments, I worried that we'd reach Cape Town before I found him. Spotting a "bed-boy" (bed-steward), I told him I was looking for Captain Phillips and could he help me? "Madam," he replied, "I only makes up beds. I don't look for men." With barely an hour to spare I found Harry alone in his compartment. Soon thereafter his traveling companion returned from the dining car to find Harry embracing a strange woman. I was quickly introduced—"I want you to meet my wife," said a slightly embarrassed Harry. "Your wife?" the soldier queried, his eyebrows raised high, and mercifully left us alone.

Durban: Health Center Practice

When World War II ended and Harry was demobilized, it no longer made sense for us to take on short-term jobs. We had to think seriously about long-term commitments and make important career decisions. We knew the kind of doctors we wanted to be: salaried family practitioners working with others to improve the health and social conditions of needy people. But we didn't know where to look for such jobs. We were attracted by what little we'd read about social medicine, and I'd been most impressed when I heard Henry Sigerist, an internationally known medical historian, speak about social medicine during his visit to the University of Cape Town. But we hadn't seen examples of social medicine practice; our knowledge of the field was purely theoretical.

Our combined South African medical experience at this time—Port Elizabeth, Umtata, Cape Town, and the army—hadn't really satisfied us; for the most part we had only been treating physical illness. So it was our good fortune that we were soon to be part of a medical practice which fitted our conviction that health and well-being stem from total life circumstances in which medical care plays an important though limited role. The work we chose to do had a lasting influence on our future actions as doctors and as people. To explain its impact I need to provide some background, medical and otherwise, of those times.

In the aftermath of World War II South Africans, like other people, felt the need to create a better world. Many leaders of the Afrikaner Nationalist Party, because of their bitter resentment of the British, had supported the Nazis, but a fair number of Afrikaners as well as English-speaking people were ready for moderate social changes. There was also a liberal minority eager for enlightened, progressive political action. This attitude of reform spilled over into the field of medical care.

Our involvement in a practice of social medicine came about through a set of events triggered by the publication and partial acceptance of a truly remarkable report.[1] In February 1942, in the South African Parliament, the Minister of Health accepted on behalf of the government a motion to appoint a commission "to investigate and recommend the best measures to be adopted for ensuring adequate health services for all sections of the population of the Union." Following this the governor-general appointed the National Health Services Commission:

to inquire into, report and advise upon—

(1) the provision of an organized National Health Service, in conformity with the modern conception of "Health," which will ensure adequate medical, dental, nursing and hospital services for *all* sections of the people of the Union of South Africa;

(2) the administrative, legislative and financial measures which would be necessary in order to provide the Union of South Africa with such a National Health Service.

Dr. Henry Gluckman, a physician member of Parliament, and a pioneer of community medicine, headed the commission and a handful of dedicated doctors worked with him in designing the national health service. They understood the importance of social factors in health and illness and recognized the deplorable conditions of South Africa's poverty-stricken rural people.

South Africa's white population, except in certain rural pockets, had reasonably good health, access to well-trained professionals, and health statistics equivalent to those in most Western countries. But in terms of numbers whites were the minority population. The majority of South Africa's people—colored, Indian, and particularly black—had inferior health, few services, and death rates like those of Third World countries.

Recommendations for organization of the National Health Service rested on two important assumptions. First, it is no longer possible for individuals working alone to give adequate attention; doctors and auxiliaries working together in teams are necessary for effective medical care. Second, the primary aim of medical practice is the promotion and maintenance of health.

The commission's blueprint guided the development of a network of health centers in neglected rural and urban areas—each center to serve the total population of its defined geographic region. Health education, prevention of illness, and treatment was to be given by a work-team of a general practitioner, family nurses, and health assistants trained as health educators. A total of four hundred centers was planned to cover the country by 1955. All personal health services (ambulatory and hospital) were to be controlled by the central Ministry of Health and financing was to come from a general health tax.

Three doctors were key to the Gluckman plans: George Gale, secretary for health and executive controller, David Landau, coordinator of all the centers, and Sidney Kark, who with his wife Emily had developed the prototype health center model in a rural Zulu community. An ardent and lifetime advocate of social medicine, Kark headed the Institute of Family and Community Health where we and like-minded colleagues practiced this new type of medical care.[2]

We learned about the health center movement indirectly. During his year in Egypt serving with the South African Medical Corps in 1945, Harry had shared his desert tent with a cousin of Emily Kark who suggested we might be interested in joining Kark after demobilization. I wrote a letter of inquiry explaining our circumstances. We were both offered jobs, and I was invited to start immediately, but we waited until Harry returned home to Cape Town and then traveled to Durban to learn more about the work and to find housing for the three of us—our David at the time was three years old.

After the war the demand for housing was intense. We could not find a suitable house in Durban for renting. As a stopgap

Kark suggested that Harry live in the officers' mess (the institute was housed in a former army hospital), and I in the nurses' quarters. And David? Perhaps he could remain with his grandmother 1200 miles away in Cape Town! It sounded like wartime all over again. No job was worth it. We declined. But, almost as if fated, on the day we were leaving, we heard about a doctor who'd decided to spend a year of study abroad and Durban became our new hometown.

South Africa being South Africa I was fascinated, as well as deeply troubled, in working with its different ethnic groups, and my interest in comparative research was aroused. The Institute had four health centers—Indian, colored, black, and white. But when we began only an Indian center was in place, treating the residents of a municipal, subsidized housing project. In the language of the day these projects were called housing schemes, but Indians referred to their project—no cynicism intended—as the Scheming House! Though suffering from poverty as abject as that of Africans, Indian culture remained an integrating, stabilizing force in urban areas, in stark contrast to the disrupted life of African families—a direct result of the migrant labor system. Although the average birth weight of Indian babies was the lowest of the four racial groups,[3] far fewer Indian than black babies died in infancy.

Besides my clinical work I was responsible for teaching and supervision in the mother and child program of the Institute, coinciding with my own special interest in babies. Indian babies were given "washed" curried vegetables (making the spice milder), almost as soon as they were given vegetables in their diet. I marveled at the extraordinary range of human baby adaptability, though animals go one better. Baby rhinos are weaned from mother's milk onto thorn bushes!

After our training period in the Indian center, and a year spent establishing a colored center, we were offered a new challenge. Kark, followed by Cassel, had set up the rural African center in Polela.[4] Now he asked us to develop the urban African Health Center. Harry was to be in charge and I the second medical officer. Fortunately, some forty years later, we still have copies of a few of our annual reports and our research publications to jog my memory. We also have a detailed later account of the Lamontville African Center—written by the doctor who took over from Harry when we left Durban in 1954—although he gave it an assumed name.[5]

I'm again embarrassed to confess how little I knew then about the history of South Africa, particularly the history of black/white relationships. It was only later that I delved seriously into historical, political, and anthropological writings, commission reports, journalists' accounts—and read every modern novel by South African authors I could lay my hands on.[6] But in 1946 I still had no clear idea of how taxation of blacks forced them into towns to earn the necessary cash or how the needs of modern industry, and particularly the development of the diamond and gold mines, enticed (and exploited) a flood of rural Africans into the towns while "influx control" tried to stem the tide by making them "temporary sojourners." Temporary residents didn't need permanent housing, or other social services, with the result that conditions in the peri-urban slums became too appalling to ignore. By 1936 more blacks lived outside the "reserves" than in them, and disease, malnutrition, prostitution, crime, alcoholism, venereal infections, and illegitimacy grew to epidemic proportions. In the 1930s a partial remedy was put in place with the construction of subsidized housing for Africans on the borders of white towns: creating regulated communities living in segregated (but sanitary) "locations" under the supervision of white government authority.[7]

The African township, Lamontville, had been established by the Durban municipality in 1934 with the construction of 182 semidetached houses built of concrete, each house consisting of a bedroom, a living-room, and a small kitchen with a wood or coal-burning stove, a sink with piped water, and a food storage area. A concrete structure in the backyard held a flush toilet and cold-water shower. Every home had a small piece of ground, front and back, in which vegetables could be grown. For many years these "Old Location" homes were the only ones with electricity and were much sought after even after newer houses were built.

A white superintendent, advised by a committee of black male residents, was responsible for the management of Lamontville, and he seemed sympathetic to the health center. I'd go with Harry to the monthly meetings of the superintendent and his advisory committee, but I never opened my mouth. Harry did all the talking about health center matters—it wasn't seemly for women in African society to discuss affairs judged to be the prerogative of men—and it was important for us to be accepted by the group. The committee was very pleased with the Lamontville Center when a group of liberal Durbanites, responding to health center staff initiatives in 1948, donated a community center as a type of living war memorial.

However simple the housing, it was far superior to the unsanitary shacks in which most Durban African (and many Indian) families lived. Our population was largely Zulu with a small number of other southern Africans and a scattering of Nyasa men married to Zulu women. Single persons were excluded; housing was intended for families only. The type of resident varied widely, from the few who'd previously lived in other municipal housing projects to those who'd come directly from rural, tribal living to a large number whose previous housing had been in slums. Few people, once resident, ever moved out, but there were an equal number of (unofficial) visitors as residents at any one time who came to look for work or for medical care. Almost all the adults were born in rural areas, but the majority of their children were born in Durban. The men worked as unskilled (a few semiskilled) laborers in the industries of greater Durban; the majority of mothers stayed at home with their children though quite a number worked as domestic servants for white families and came back to their own families at night. But some who slept in special quarters provided in the backyards of employers' homes returned only on their days off and Sundays.

Our clientele reflected the background of our population. Their housing in Lamontville was sanitary, but many people brought with them the unhealthy consequences of malnutrition and medical neglect, as well as the infestations common to lives disrupted by separation of families and extremely unhygienic environmental conditions. Added to this was the emotional effect of living in a constantly expanding setting, too new to fuse the heterogeneous population into a cohesive community.

We saw our first Lamontville patient in February 1948. Though at first we introduced ourselves only to the people living closest to the center, our practice soon encompassed the entire Old Location; by the end of 1949, 682 homes in three areas of Lamontville were served, 1359 by mid-1953—the practice expanding each year as more and more houses were built.

The trust we sought had to be earned and didn't come easily. We were all employed by the government, and Africans, who already mistrusted official agencies, had additional reasons for caution. Not long before we opened the Center a mobile van appeared with miniature X-ray equipment to screen the residents for tuberculosis. Those whose X rays showed the possibility of disease were given more tests and if the diagnosis was confirmed they were shipped off to TB hospitals. People suspected us of being TB officers (whom they greatly feared) though a few weeks went by before we uncovered the special reason for their suspicion. It so happened that our eye-testing chart had "confirmed" our duplicity: the second line read "T B."

Some residents doubted our ability as healers. In contrast with their diviners who knew the diagnosis without asking questions, we asked too many. Our staff, particularly the health assistants, also wanted to know too much: how many people lived in the house? what age and sex were they? what visitors were staying in the house? what did the occupants earn? how much did they spend? and on and on. Expenditure always exceeded disclosed income, extra money coming mainly from the sale of illegally brewed homemade beer. Perhaps we would inform the police?

It was a great day for me when I was given the recipe for making this brew.

We soon learned which illnesses predominated. Children under two suffered from acute respiratory ailments, ear infections, pneumonias, and diarrheas. Some signs of malnutrition were present in all babies when breast milk alone became insufficient nourishment or after weaning. In our first year of practice in Lamontville we saw many cases of gross malnutrition—kwashiorkor, pellagra, rickets—but later such cases were limited to the children of rural visitors or newly arrived residents. Subclinical primary tuberculosis was common, and skin rashes were frequent in infants. Scabies, impetigo, and tropical ulcers usually affected preschool and school-age children. Parasitic diseases like schistosomiasis were most common in school-age children, but worm infestations of all types, especially roundworms, were almost universal after infancy. After we asked for detailed descriptions, mothers took to bringing or sending children with large jars filled with worms—a kind of show and tell which made me feel squeamish.

We found it useless to separate promotion of health, prevention, and cure; medicinal treatment without health education was hopeless. The houses had flush toilets, but because adults didn't believe children's feces could be harmful, small children defecated freely in the yards surrounding the houses, and unwashed hands contaminated food. One of our colleagues, only half in jest, suggested that on prearranged days we should hand out worm medicine to the entire township at one go. He didn't say what we should do with the results. At times measles and whooping cough were epidemic. In adults amoebic dysentery, venereal diseases, alcoholism, burns, and other injuries were frequent, but tuberculosis was the main cause of death.

Slowly the people we served got to know and trust us—helped by the fact that aside from the doctors all our staff were Africans, some of whom lived in Lamontville. Luckily, antibiotics (developed during the war) helped to establish our credibility; during our first three weeks of practice we cured a young child desperately ill from bacterial pneumonia and later proved our ability to cure venereal disease. Just as important was our obvious fondness for our patients, especially the babies. (For years after I came to the United States, I found white babies pale and anemic-looking, not nearly as attractive as the curly-headed, big-eyed black babies—before they became malnourished.) It was useful, too, that we learned the African names for some ailments, for it showed we understood their sicknesses, though we treated them differently than their indigenous healers did. We pleased the community also by keeping sick people at home in bed whenever possible rather than sending them to a hospital. Our staff was stable: the same team of nurse and doctor worked together in the center seeing the same families that they visited in the field, and our health educators had a similar continuing relationship with families—my model for later work.

Many of the residents of Lamontville believed that misfortunes of all kinds, bad health and failure in general, were due to the action of evildoers—people who were angry with them or jealous of their success, beauty, fertility, etc. Misfortune might result, too, from the action of ancestors displeased by the breaking of taboos or deviation from customary traditions and ancestral respect. In circumstances like these treatment by Western-trained doctors wasn't relevant for we couldn't divine who the ill wisher was or what he'd used that caused the symptoms. Nor did we know what medications would be effective against the poisons or what sacrifices would assuage the ancestors. Such situations called for the ministrations of the *inyanga* (African herbalist) or *isangoma* (diviner). But most residents distinguished between illnesses for which we could do little, and illnesses such as "town diseases"—primarily sexual diseases—for which we could do a lot. I was delighted when an *inyanga* sent one of his seven wives to me for treatment of her venereal infection.

There were times when we shared our patients with the indigenous healers. As people got to know us better, some patients came to us with emotional disturbances like *fufunyana* (a complex syndrome due to spirits or demons which possess the victim), after African traditional treatment had failed. A young girl who lived a long distance from us, in Zululand, came for consultation, accompanied by an older relative who told me the girl was suffering from *fufunyana*. Lengthy questioning revealed that the girl had been ill for six months and was steadily getting worse. Her worried father had sent her to several *izinyanga* (herbalists) and *izangoma* (diviners) with no improvement. Her symptoms were weakness, a disinclination for food, loss of weight, and episodes of bizarre behavior due to "a spirit which took possession of her," dictated her actions, and spoke through her in foreign tongues. This illness began shortly after the father had arranged for her to marry an elderly man of his acquaintance. The girl, powerless to resist her father, shyly admitted in response to my gentle probing that she preferred a young man she'd known for several years. When my examination showed no physical cause for her illness, I didn't argue about the diagnosis of *fufunyana*, but told them I believed the spirit didn't want the girl to marry the old man; a younger man would be better. Nutritional advice, a placebo, and assurance that the girl would get better very soon—if they followed my instructions—ended the visit. Some months later I saw another patient from the same area sent to me by the family of the first girl. She had recovered completely and was happily married to her young man.

Another time the chief wife of a subchief arrived with his third and newest wife, much younger than herself. They were both clad in traditional dress, blanketed and beaded, and with elaborate hairdos. I no longer recall the diagnosis, but after the young wife had been examined and treated, I was surprised to find the chief wife waiting for me. We spoke through the health center family nurse, whose many duties included that of interpreter. (Our knowledge of Zulu, like that of Xhosa, was quite inadequate.) I was told that the young wife was already the favorite of the husband; my medicine would make her stronger and even more desirable. If *she* was given good medicine, the first wife wanted some too. A reasonable enough argument I thought and complied.

Harry had a middle-aged patient, a truck driver with *umeqo*,[8] manifesting itself through chronic ulceration on the backs of both hands. His condition, the man explained, was produced by one of his fellow-workers who had put medicine on the steering wheel of his truck so he wouldn't be able to hold down his very desirable job and the other man's brother would get his position. The medical diagnosis was leprosy; fortunately the patient agreed to a period of treatment in a leprosarium and later returned home cured. In a very similar case, a man who had contact with a telephone at his place of work became ill through *muti* (medicine) supposedly placed on the handle of the telephone.

I don't remember hearing any African women complaining of having too many children—so many died in infancy and children were highly valued—but many women came because of infertility. One of Harry's barren patients developed pseudocyesis (false pregnancy). After waiting many months for the baby to be born, she reported to him that she'd been bewitched and had given birth to a *likkewaan* (a type of lizard) which ran away before anyone had a chance to capture it. This was her way of saving face.

All too often we saw the impact of South Africa's inhuman political and economic policies on the lives of individual patients. Illegitimacy, rare in traditional rural Zulu society, was rampant in Durban. In Lamontville illegitimacy had become a serious problem for young girls—to be expected since the municipality had built a six-story barracks to house single men on the outskirts of the township. These men came from the tribal reserves under contract to work for short periods in industry and many spent their evenings in the township drinking home-brewed beer. Mothers made extra money this way, but at the same time illegitimate births increased among their daughters. One day Mrs. Nguni came to me for aid.

"Udokotela must help me."
"If I can. What's the trouble?"

"Barbara is soon coming home from the Mission Boarding School for the long school holidays. I have to go to my job in town and she will get pregnant. Udokotela must help me. I don't know what to do."

I had no ready answer either. For a while we both sat, brows furrowed, thinking hard. What could I do? The pill hadn't yet been invented; mechanical types of contraception weren't suitable for a virgin. Abstinence seemed to be the answer, but how to assure it? At last I made a tentative suggestion. I would personally employ Barbara during the holidays; she could act as my scribe. The photocopier hadn't been invented either, or if it had, certainly our little library didn't have one. Mrs. Nguni was delighted and neither one of us asked Barbara's opinion. Each morning at 8:30 Mrs. Nguni brought Barbara to my office; each afternoon at 5:30 I handed her back to her mother's safekeeping. In the interim Barbara, a thin, rather silent and repressed sixteen-year-old, sat quietly, day after day, hour after hour, slowly copying the articles I wanted out of the big, bound volumes of journals I had requested from distant medical libraries. I didn't dare ask her if she enjoyed the work—it must have been deadly dull—but I paid her well. By the time I left Durban I'd accumulated many boxes of reprints of articles relevant to my research on infant growth—which I most reluctantly discarded when we left for Boston. In disposing of these papers I came across several in Barbara's neat, clear longhand. I recall, even now, that the first copy was of an article in *Human Biology*—an excellent journal though hardly light reading even for the interested researcher. Thankfully, Barbara hadn't become pregnant, and I'd found out that she wanted to study to be a nursery schoolteacher. Mrs. Nguni, who earned her living as a domestic servant, hadn't been keen on a further period of Barbara's dependency, but she was persuaded.

Little Jantjies was a more desperate case. His father Kleinbooi, a colored man, worked as a cleaner at our Institute at government wage rates for an unskilled laborer. Kleinbooi lived with a black woman, somewhat mentally retarded, in a shack they'd fashioned from an abandoned fowl run. Jantjies, a sickly, underfed baby, developed kwashiorkor on weaning. Home visits, health education, and milk powder all proved ineffective, and we decided the only way to save little Jantjies' life was to admit him to a hospital for a period of intensive care. Two possibilities were open to us: King Edward Hospital, one of the largest in all of Africa, was the black Provincial hospital. Care there was free, but the hospital of 1200 beds (now 2000) was always overcrowded, with two children to a cot and extra mattresses on the floor. McCords Zulu Hospital, an American Board Mission hospital—situated in the middle of a white residential area to the great annoyance of most area residents—was a private hospital and required payment, small though that was. Care at McCords was excellent, but there was no way Kleinbooi could pay for it. Harry and I decided it was Jantjies' only chance and paid the bills ourselves. The child did beautifully in the hospital but gradually regressed at home. This cycle was repeated several times before he passed the most vulnerable age of infancy, and we were satisfied he could survive at home under close health center supervision. I remember once standing with Harry outside the Kleinbooi shack while Harry tried to show Mrs. Kleinbooi by the position of the sun in the sky how often she should give Jantjies food.

Fortunately for the family and our sanity, one of our medical colleagues discovered that married employees got an extra cost of living allowance from the government. She told Kleinbooi he'd be much better off if he got legally married. Since he had no idea how to get a license, she did all the preliminaries, and on the day of the civil marriage she took the couple (and Jantjies) in her car to the court and witnessed the wedding. I often look at the beaded necklace and belt given to me by Kleinbooi and remember little Jantjies.

I still recall with great pleasure the beautiful care lavished on the first-born infant of one of our best-educated mothers. She and I both delighted in looking at her baby's weekly weight gain recorded on his growth chart; she brought him every week even though it wasn't really necessary, missing only one week in fifty-two when our session coincided with her history exam. (She was studying to become a teacher.) One week the infant developed diarrhea and though I didn't show my worry I was almost as anxious as the mother. I insisted on a second opinion from a somewhat surprised colleague—the case was no different from others I saw every day alone. The baby made an uneventful recovery, and I realized that too close an attachment to a patient can cloud professional judgment. But it's difficult to be detached when frequent contact makes for bonding between doctor and patient.

African mothers breast-fed their babies freely, both for nourishment and comfort, but when a baby developed the syndrome of frequent, green, watery stools, and dehydration that spelled the dreaded *Inyoni*,[9] it was abruptly weaned. An *inyanga* was consulted in such cases to confirm the diagnosis and to validate the mother's belief that an ill wisher had put *muti* on the path she had walked on, thus making her milk toxic and causing the baby's symptoms. The *inyanga* would prescribe purges, enemas, and, worst of all, weaning the baby from the "poisoned" breast milk. We lost many babies that way. Sometimes mothers would come to us when they saw that the *inyanga's* cure wasn't working, and though I didn't dispute the diagnosis I managed at times to persuade mothers to resume breast-feeding. Once I got a baby back on the breast three weeks after weaning!—and the baby recovered.

I've emphasized the tragic aspects of African urban life, but of course there was pleasure, humor, and comedy also—African society had all the complexities of human societies everywhere. Not surprisingly, certain aspects of culture, like ethnic jokes, needed a relatively long period of intimacy and trust before they could be shared with people from a very different background. Our team meetings became times of very frank discussion and camaraderie—no wonder the white janitor, a Pretoria stooge who spied on us, reported the shocking behavior of white

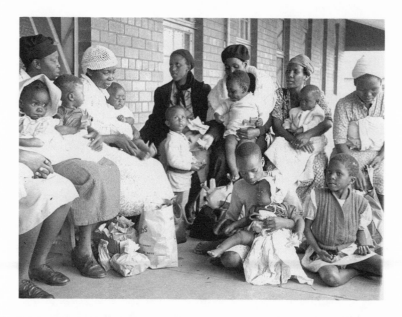

Lamontville mother-and-baby clinic

women who gave cigarettes to black men and allowed them to smoke in their presence at these meetings.

At one such meeting a health assistant told the following story: Emily Molefe and her husband, Simon, were living happily together until the arrival from Polela of Albert Mkize who'd found work in the same chrome factory that employed Simon. The two men became friends, and Simon, a hospitable man, often took Albert home with him to enjoy Emily's delicious home brew. Frequent contact roused mutual desire. How to arrange their meetings? Emily solved this problem with what I thought of as Boccaccian ingenuity. Every morning Simon went off to the factory in his tattered work clothes, battered hat on head, and lunch in his old tin box. Hidden inside the hatband lining was a note from Emily to Albert. Every evening, Simon arrived home in the same clothes, hat on head, empty lunch box in hand. Inside the hat band was a note from Albert to Emily.

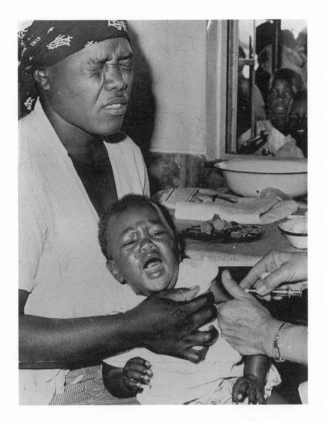

Sharing the pain

Amusing stories and warm memories of individual patients and their successful treatment were very important for our morale, but more so was the improvement in community health. By 1949 we had reduced infant mortality to 65 deaths in the first year of life per 1,000 live births, when at the same time the overall rate for Durban African infants was 369 per 1,000! (The latter figure is of course exaggerated because many births which didn't occur in hospitals went unregistered while burial required a death certificate.) All the same, our accurate count showed what could be done. Another important index was satisfactory growth. By our second year of practice Lamontville babies were, on average, a pound heavier at age one year than the babies who had previously attended the local municipal clinic. Our success was due to regular examinations, health education, immunizations, nutritional advice, and the use of dried skim milk powder, one of our most effective medicines. When patients were underfed, food, rather than medicine, was the appropriate remedy. The Government Health Department provided us with a supply of skim milk for medicinal purposes, but drew the line at full cream milk, a food.

The Institute acted as a magnet, attracting compassionate Durbanites—mostly women—who volunteered their services. The Union of Jewish Women of Durban gave the health center a monthly donation for doctors to order food for malnourished babies. I had the satisfying duty of examining the weekly growth charts, picking out the babies who hadn't been thriving, and prescribing for them eggs, fruit, full cream milk, vegetables, and other necessary foods. Union members then bought, packaged, and distributed the supplements to the mothers of these babies at the special weekly sessions we arranged. There were times when a mother stayed away and sent a young child to collect the baby's food; we knew the food was shared with older siblings, but the effect on infants was still obvious in terms of weight gain and generally improved health.

The Lamont Government Primary School gave formal education to the children of the township up to Std. 7. But volunteers supplied additional opportunities. A Durban College Women's Guild ran a preschool for one hundred Lamontville children, and Lamont Community Center volunteers provided adult literacy classes, a library, a debating society, physical training, and sporting facilities for Lamontville youth. This center also acted as a bridge between old and disabled people and children needing welfare services and the official welfare agencies of Durban.

Health education was our long-term strategy for improving community health. We did our best to learn about illness as viewed by patients and their families and tried hard to teach about health in a way which fitted patients' cultural patterns. This kind of education can be illustrated in the home care of sick patients.[10]

In 1951, during six consecutive months, detailed records were kept of 108 patients getting home nursing care, all of whom in the absence of this service would have been sent to hospital for admission. There are many advantages to this type of care. The family nurse sees her patient not in temporary hospital surroundings, unrelated to the development of the disease, but in the same environment which gives rise to the illness. The person in the home, chosen by the nurse to care for the patient under supervision, is receptive to an educational experience which raises her and the family's standard of health at that time and in the future. In a case of infectious illness she is taught the possible sources of that infection and how to prevent its spread; in nutritional disease she learns the dietary deficiencies likely to be responsible and the foods needed for maintaining health. Treatment of a patient at home is psychologically easier, especially for a child, where the tensions and fears of a strange place aren't added to the physical burdens of the illness. Treatment at home also costs less and helps to build family and community knowledge and self-reliance.

Our family nurses, trained in midwifery as well as in general care, kept a register of all pregnant women in Lamontville, most of whom they persuaded to attend the health center for regular prenatal care. Before our center opened the majority of deliveries were done by two "granny midwives" who lived in the area and received instruction from the Durban Department of Public Health before being licensed by them. One was very fat and short, the other very thin and somewhat taller—an incongruous-looking pair—but efficient and well liked by the residents. The "grannys" continued in their work but were now under the direct supervision of our experienced family nurses.

Only the director of nursing at the Institute was white. All the rest of the nurses were black—wonderfully warm, solid, patient, motherly figures—the real primary care workers of the

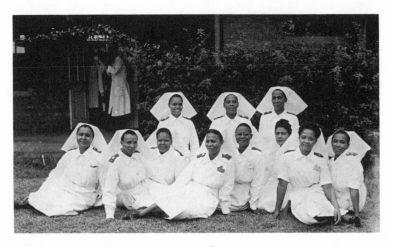

Family nurses: The real primary care workers

Institute. I remember after 1952, when the Nationalist Party again came into power and we endlessly debated our future in South Africa, Harry would tell me we *had* to leave. He anticipated an inevitable bloody confrontation based on color. In such a clash he couldn't bear to be on the side opposing people the likes of Sister Makanya, Mzimela, Ngcobo—family nurses at the health center and our good friends.

We were of course learning as much as teaching, and our teaching wasn't confined to patients. The Institute was a training center; all staff took part in the training through lectures, team discussions, community group meetings, and research. One colleague trained health assistants to be laboratory technicians; a staff statistician taught another group of health assistants to be record clerks. The Institute was fortunate to have a distinguished anthropologist and an accomplished psychologist on its staff. One physician devoted attention to the field of family dynamics, another to nutrition, yet another to adolescence; I became knowledgeable in infant, and Harry in preschool, growth patterns.

We kept detailed records on the population of Lamontville: their numbers, ethnicity, religion, home languages, deaths in each age group, and the diseases from which they died, the many illnesses of the living, immunizations of the children, etc. The median income per family per month between 1949 and 1950 was twelve pounds, five shillings, and fourpence, but this did not include illegal earnings from home brew. As a first step in health education to improve nutrition in the community, our health assistants conducted a survey of the foods commonly produced and consumed in Lamontville. Pregnant women, infants, and preschool children received special attention. My own research interests focused on comparative infant growth.

How does a health service deal with problems of the magnitude we faced and not give up in despair? We were buoyed partly by the optimism and stamina of our youth, partly by the strength of others who believed in the rightness of what we were all doing, and partly by the excitement of learning how another culture viewed the world. It was often exhausting, often very sad, but never dull work. And there were moments of triumph for each of us, some of which I have mentioned earlier.

But what of our own children through this period of service to other people's families? Household help was plentiful and inexpensive, but the psychological, emotional conflicts remained. I didn't work in David's infancy. His first year we spent in Ladysmith, Natal, where Harry was attached to a South African military base hospital. During David's second year, when Harry went to Egypt, he and I returned to Cape Town—happily sharing a bedroom in my parents' home. It was then that I became a student in public health at the University of Cape Town and employed Katy, a middle-aged colored woman recommended to me by her aunt—a fine and gentle woman whom I knew well. Katy remained with us until we left South Africa.

Katy had grown up in a rural, Moravian-mission community and believed in the Bible as written. She was a marvelous nurse with each baby in its early dependent stage and guarded the children like a mother lioness, but she had a rigid, authoritarian personality. We often differed on how children should behave;

Katy believing that children must *never* contradict adults—at least not to their faces. We disagreed also on what caused illness. To Katy bare feet on a cold concrete surface spelled pneumonia. Drinking cold water when sweating from the heat had equally dire results. The fact that we were doctors was irrelevant to Katy and the children alike. Faced with a choice the children usually obeyed Katy. When Rosalie at three asked me who God was and I began to explain, she cut me short with "I think Katy's God."

Harry and I treated Katy with great respect. On one occasion, when traveling with her and our three children by car to Cape Town, the hotel where we'd planned to spend a night refused to take Katy. Furious, we refused to stay there ourselves and all of us spent an uncomfortable night in the car—each sleeping child resting his or her head on the lap of an adult. I remember how, in an act of derision and defiance, I emptied Rosalie's potty in the market square where we'd parked for the night. But I didn't feel the warm affection for Katy that I felt for Sakkie—nor she for me. I was the mother whom she regarded as her rival, and she referred to me as "his mother" or "her mother." She adored "her children" and was very proud of their achievements, though she seldom praised them directly. Harry jokes sometimes, telling people we had to leave South Africa to free ourselves of Katy.

Harry and I started work together in Durban and, except for the three precious months of maternity leave, I wasn't at home with Mark during infancy as I had been with David. Fortunately, I was working at the colored center at the time and that was very close to our house. Even more fortunate was the fact that Mark, from the beginning, was what people called a "good child." Since he was extraordinarily patient and uncomplaining, and babies quickly learn to adapt, we evolved a nursing schedule to suit me during working hours and to suit Mark outside those hours. I fed him before leaving for work, during my lunch hour, and very hurriedly during my afternoon tea break, working on health center records at night to make up the time; after working hours I nursed him on demand. But I was unhappy to be away from him so soon and when I was pregnant with Rosalie three years later I began to dread the prospect of not being home with yet another child. During that pregnancy Sidney Kark asked me if I'd be interested in pursuing my infant growth studies in greater depth. "Yes," I replied, but thought no more about it until Rosalie was born. As with Mark, so with Rosalie, I worked until almost the day before labor in order to keep those three months of maternity leave intact. During that time I decided to resign and told Sidney my intention to do so.

It was a most upsetting interview. Sidney said the research proposal he'd sent in for me had been granted the previous day; he felt it would reflect very badly on the Institute if the grant were to be returned. It's difficult to appreciate my dilemma without some understanding of the atmosphere in which we operated. We were a closely knit group akin, I often thought, to secular missionaries. Many of the senior staff, particularly Sidney, were deadly serious and single-minded in their mission. They lived and breathed health center ideology, leaving little room for the "selfishness" of a private life. There was no way I could let Sidney and the Institute down, but I desperately wanted to be with my children. My solution was to accept the bursary from the Council for Scientific and Industrial Research provided my office could be in my house. The compromise was accepted. My clinical work at Lamontville became only sporadic as occasionally I relieved colleagues on vacation or sick leave. My teaching duties continued and my interest in the mother and baby program remained, but I was no longer directly responsible for the lives and needs of people in Lamontville. I was home when I needed to be, I had a wonderful research associate, and I had far more time with my children.

Most of us were working couples (doctor-doctor, doctor-nurse, doctor-dentist) with heavy responsibilities, but patients' problems, not staff difficulties, were discussed at the Institute. In looking back, however, I know that many of us had personal problems that needed strong collegial support. "Missionaries," however, are not encouraged to share their own dilemmas at work, and we were expected to be role models for new trainees. Every doctor and nurse accepted into the health center system spent six months of orientation at the Institute, much of his or her time under the tutelage of clinicians like Harry and me, or our equivalents at the other health centers established at the Institute and at Polela. After their apprenticeship they joined health centers already set up or started new ones in places preselected nationally as areas of great need.

From our early days we had physician trainees attached to us. Each trainee was given a certain number of families to look after, as well as one family to study in depth over the entire six-month period. I will always enjoy the image of one of these doctors sitting with a young African baby on his knee and in his booming voice gleefully singing, "Baa baa black sheep." One young trainee became a father soon after arrival in Durban. Every week he'd report to me: "I know everything about a baby of one week"; "I know everything about a baby of two weeks." One of our trainees became so important to his assigned family during his six months as their special doctor that ever after that the family reckoned time by him: "That was before our doctor came," or "That was while our doctor was here," or "That was after our doctor left."

These physician trainees were no run-of-the-mill people. One, a cultured Englishman, ex-Indian army, was the first person who introduced us to recordings of Bartok's music. Another young doctor, with whom Harry became fast friends, was an Afrikaner liberal, a position more difficult to maintain than if he had been of British stock or Jewish. He died of a heart attack at twenty-nine, and we gave his name to our third son. One trainee, who distinguished himself during World War II in Burma and received the Order of the British Empire, started the industrial center of the Institute. And another, an artist as well as a doctor, married our personal physician, thereby creating a double bond between us.

We formed deep attachments with several of our colleagues, and many members of the group have stayed in touch. Even if our shared experience turned out to be shorter than we all had intended, it remained with us and had a deep influence on our future work and behavior. When the movement toward a national health service was obviously doomed, and South Africa was drifting toward becoming a police state, most of us emigrated—to Israel (following Sidney and Emily Kark), the United States, Britain, Canada, or Australia. Almost without exception, we chose not to enter the private practice of clinical medicine. The majority of us became teachers, administrators, epidemiologists, health educators, or practitioners in the field of public health or community medicine.

Most doctors even today think of health only in terms of diseases for which curative and preventive clinical services must be provided. But the years we spent in Durban, as practitioners of social medicine, taught us that health and health care must also be seen in the light of historical, political, economic, and sociocultural circumstances. Medicine alone cannot cure the illnesses caused by racial discrimination with its accompanying low wages, malnutrition, bad housing, unhealthy sanitation, and social disruption. Nowhere is this more apparent than in the shocking death rates of young black children—inexact as the figures may be.

It's difficult to measure the effect of a particular philosophy of practice, but I believe the work made possible by Dr. Gluckman and put into practice by Kark and his followers who worked in the movement—short though its life was—had a forceful impact on the thinking and practice of the countries they entered.[11] For example, America's neighborhood health centers, which came into being as part of the "War on Poverty" of the 1960s, were modeled directly on the South African pattern.[12]

Perhaps the most painful, emotional, and rewarding hours of our lives came in our final parting with the staff and people of Lamontville. Sister Mzimela, though a Christian, sacrificed a goat to her ancestors to ensure our safety. The black staff and the people of the township gave us a farewell party. We sat on the platform in the community hall while they made speeches—I suppose we made some too, but I don't recall them. Hymns were sung for us while I wept unashamedly, and they brought us gifts. Mine were a handmade, clay, decorated beer pot of a type used at communal beer-drinking feasts, a beaded necklace, a few shillings of hard earned money to buy food for our journey, a live fowl, a bucket of lichees, and a few papayas. For Harry a Zulu shield topped with leopard skin as befits a front rank warrior, given with the words that it was for "A white man with a black heart."

At the end they presented both of us with two framed scrolls. One was from the black staff—it pains me yet that they referred to themselves as "the non-European staff," but that was the custom then—the other from "the residents of the Lamontville Native Location." They thanked us, remembered their early suspicion and their later trust, told us how they appreciated our efforts, and ended with "Siya Ni Bonga" (We praise you).

I carefully put these treasures away. Though some jobs have come very close, none other has given Harry or me quite the same feeling of "rightness" in what we were doing.

Cape Town: 1954

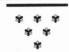

In 1952, during his year of study for his diploma in public health, Harry learned about a most unusual and progressive student movement. Medical students had started free evening clinics in the Cape Flats for people living in makeshift dumps only a few miles from the University of Cape Town (UCT).

I write here about the growth of these clinics, not only for the part that Harry, later, played in them, but because involvement in the clinics over the last forty years has been a unique educational experience for the students of UCT. I also want to show how a university encouraged its students to care for people less privileged than themselves. Understandably, good things about South Africa are seldom reported in the overseas press, but even in South Africa, outside of Cape Town, few people know about this progressive humanitarian student program. I believe it's important to record this activity: the impression that *all* South African whites are evil and racist is inaccurate and unjust.

These shanty townships were not only deficient in sanitation, housing, and water supplies, but were also regularly flooded during heavy winter rains. Until World War II the Cape Flats was an area where colored people lived as well as a few poor white families. But when industry burgeoned with the war, a stream of Africans came looking for work in Cape Town. While most were placed in nearby housing projects, including the unconscionable barracks for "single" men, many settled (illegally) in the bush and sand of the Cape Flats or in semideveloped districts like Windermere and nearby Kensington.

Residents of the Flats put up *pondokkies*, using random scraps of abandoned materials: corrugated iron, cardboard, pieces of wood, old cans, and discarded sacks. So noxious was this environment that deaths from tuberculosis increased alarmingly, but until the war had ended the municipality didn't have the funds for adequate slum clearance and rebuilding.

Private organizations and individuals responded to these reports of misery, among them the Union of Jewish Women who set up a soup kitchen in Kensington in 1943 and almost immediately began an alliance with the UCT students which still exists more than forty years later. The volunteer directly responsible for starting the clinics was a medical student who spent his summer vacation driving an ambulance to earn his tuition fees. One of the areas he happened to visit was Windermere. Deeply shocked by the extent of poverty and the lack of medical care he saw, he began a crusade to start a student-run free clinic in the area. In this he was supported by Dr. Golda Selzer, a pathologist at the medical school and wife of our teacher Dr. Frank Forman. But, for many years, keeping the clinic going was an uphill struggle.

The first clinic began in mid-July of 1943 on a Friday night— traditionally a drinking night for laborers after getting their weekly pay—and eight people came. The following Friday there were fifty. Patients were seen in the quite inadequate premises of an African Methodist Episcopal school which had no running water, only dim lighting, and little storage space. Still, clinics continued each week regardless of weather, transportation problems, and university examinations. Students who couldn't get rides took a bus and walked through the bush. When patients were too ill to come, students trudged through the area to see them in their shacks. Their spirits remained high while they gathered equipment and supplies and found volunteer staff to be their preceptors.

For many years university students had collected money for hospitals—mainly for the support of indigent patients—at an annual Mardi-Gras type Hospital Rag. When the Province took over the financing of voluntary hospitals, the great bulk of Rag funds went to the clinics.

A few student leaders had broad visions for the future of their clinics. They saw them becoming not only health and welfare service centers, but also community development centers, and they discussed these ideas with Dr. Davie, the principal of UCT in 1948. His feelings about the social responsibility of a university went far beyond those of his predecessors.

Dr. Davie insisted that the university as a whole had a responsibility for such a program. And he wanted *all* students, not just medical, to take part in this project—a joint health and welfare center of the university, but under student leadership. In 1956 the South African historian, De Kiewiet, then president of the University of Rochester, spoke of Dr. Tom Davie as "The most outstanding personality in South African university life . . . the profile of courage itself." [1]

Officially recognized and registered as a welfare organization in 1954, SHAWCO (Students Health and Welfare Centres Organization) planned its expansion—including the appointment of a physician as a Senior Lecturer in Social Medicine. Half of this person's time would be devoted to supervising the medical students at clinic sessions and advising the health committee on ways to improve the health of the Windermere citizens.

Harry was offered this job and began his work in January 1954. His heart was in the student project because of the time he had already spent serving impoverished communities in Durban, and he knew what he wanted to accomplish. Besides supervising the evening treatment clinics, he soon introduced preventive services by starting child care and prenatal daytime sessions. His next step was to encourage a family and social orientation toward health and illness. To carry this through, he assigned selected Windermere families to volunteer students who became health advisers to these families. Some students took this responsibility lightly, but others became forceful advocates for their families, going to great lengths to get them what they needed and spending extended periods of time with them.

In time SHAWCO took over social services in Windermere, an action which added heavy responsibility to students and staff.

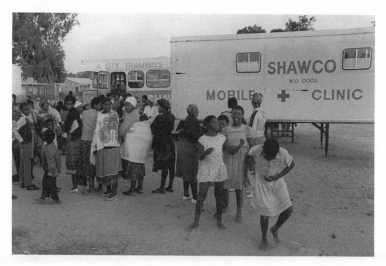

SHAWCO *mobile clinic*

A director of welfare services was appointed, for SHAWCO was then responsible for all the family welfare, regular casework, and twenty-four-hour, round-the-clock emergency services. It was also responsible for the operation of water taps. At this time area people bought their water from water-cart-sellers or collected it from municipal standpipes whose faucets were often damaged until SHAWCO hired residents to protect and manage the standpipes. Later, students began to show their concern for the elderly and disabled by operating a meals-on-wheels service—the first of its kind in South Africa.

All this work was going on while the Nationalist government was steadily implementing its demonic segregation policies through measures like the Group Areas Act. Increasingly, Africans were being removed from Windermere to areas bureaucratically designated for blacks. In response students began to provide services to outlying black areas through the use of mobile clinics.

Looking back, we see that SHAWCO students—energetic, generous, and warm-hearted though they were—were not yet

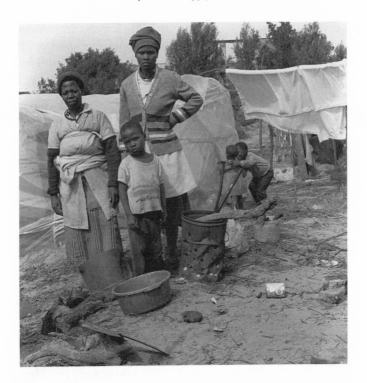

Crossroads in 1984

politicized. But their movement continued to grow. Already in
the early sixties, 75 percent of all medical students at UCT were
involved in the clinics, and students in nursing, law, sociology,
and other departments of the university were also very active.
Our latest available SHAWCO report of 1984–85 shows more than
eight hundred students participating.

When the government threatened to bulldoze the Crossroads
camp—using the danger of an outbreak of communicable disease
as an excuse—some students deflected the plan by immunizing
the squatters. That was the beginning of SHAWCO's Crossroads'
clinic. Americans were shocked into awareness of Crossroads'
existence when they saw the horror scenes of its final destruction
on their television sets.

Cape Town in 1954 was a wonderful city for children—at least white children—to grow up in. The climate was mild, without the enervating heat and humidity of Durban, or the (later) snows of Boston. The ocean was nearby and warm enough to bathe in a good part of the year; white sand beaches stretched for miles; the mountain was a majestic guardian of the city; picnic spots were plentiful; there were no traffic jams; the pace was leisurely, the cost of living low, household help easy to get.

What was I doing while Harry worked at UCT? Philip, our fourth child, was born in Cape Town about five months after we arrived there, and, as usual, I looked for a job that would satisfy me while fitting in with my family's needs.

I had resolved not to get into any more painful mother/doctor conflicts like the one I had when Mark was born, so I had absolutely no intention of looking for a full-time job. My aim was to work on the research data I had accumulated in Durban—the South African Council for Scientific and Industrial Research had extended my scholarship for a fourth year. But I did, also, accept a part-time position for two years as medical officer to the women students of the University of Cape Town.

As I recall it, that job was not a strenuous one. In fact I believe it was the first job I held in which I felt pleasantly relaxed and at ease. Young women who thought they needed a medical examination or who wanted to consult with me on personal problems made individual appointments to see me, but I was seldom faced with severe physical or emotional problems. Most of the students I saw were likable young women, fresh out of high school, and shy to disclose any emotional difficulties.

After a while I tried to get them talking more freely by telling them I'd learned that young freshmen at the university had three special problems during their first semester. Since for many it was their first time away from home, it was only natural that some felt rather lonely and homesick. Others who weren't used to concentrated study found it hard to discipline themselves to the work routine and were afraid of failing exams. And because there were now no parents to watch over boy-girl relationships, some young women weren't sure how to handle this new-found freedom. Did they perhaps have any one of these three problems? And, if so, would they like to talk to me about it? Usually this approach worked, allowing them to express their anxiety and me to reassure them.

I enjoyed the easy, leisurely contacts I had with students— appealing to my motherly instincts. But, as a doctor wanting to help communities, I directed most of my work energy into my research in South African infant growth. So, though I was living and working in Cape Town, my mind was largely focused on Durban, and what I now report adds substantial information to what I have already given on the four ethnic groups with whom we were concerned at the Institute of Family and Community Health. For more than a year I analyzed and interpreted my Durban data, presenting the results in the form of a thesis for the doctor of medicine (M.D.) degree. It seemed a perfect time for me to get the degree before we left to face an uncertain future in another country; Harry made the same decision a little later than I did. In his thesis he reviewed the racial and economic circumstances of the white and colored peoples of Cape Town and compared their public health experiences over a span of fifty years.[2] It was important for both of us to have this degree because to most Americans only M.D.'s are doctors.[3]

I began to do research in 1950 and continued to carry out research projects the rest of my professional life. As far as possible all my investigations were socially oriented: comparing access to medical care between more privileged and less fortunate people, contrasting the health of the better-off with the poor, emphasizing the prevention of illness, and looking for ways to improve the health of easily forgotten people.

Before I wrote this chapter, I reread the preface to my thesis, curious to see what my stated goals had been thirty years earlier. The language was simple, the intent clear. I had noted that the four main ethnic groups in South Africa—European, Colored, Bantu, and Indian—differed widely in their social, economic, and cultural background and that they presented a unique opportunity for comparative research. I suggested that growth in infancy could be used as an index of health and of the standard of living of the different population groups. But, if growth were also to be used as a measure of improvement or deterioration in infant health, it was necessary first to create basic South African growth curves instead of relying on U.S. and British figures. My study included birth weights, growth in the first ten days of life, and growth in the first year. In mothers I looked at success or failure in breast-feeding and the proportion of babies born in or out of wedlock.[4]

Apart from the excitement of designing and organizing this study, and the joy of completing the task, the three years spent in the actual collection of the data (in Durban) were often sheer drudgery. I'll never forget the tedium of collecting the weights of babies in their first ten days of life. As one part of this study, for eight months I, myself, weighed every healthy Bantu baby born in McCords Zulu Hospital each day, until discharge from hospital seven to ten days later.

It was essential in doing these daily weighings that I be consistent and accurate. To keep alert I played games with myself. In the "weight guessing game" I predicted each weight before actually weighing the infant and got to be pretty good at it. Such skills are easily gained and just as easily lost. The "personality game" was more fun. Each baby was different in its reaction to being undressed and placed on a cold scale. I liked to guess how passive or how unwilling each infant would be and the way in which its face, voice, and body movement would express its acceptance or outrage. The babies' mothers loved this communal weighing, undressed their infants, placed them on the scale, and waited eagerly to hear that day's weight, but after the first month or two for me the charm had worn thin.

Five hundred and ninety-eight (598) babies in all—about 5000 weighings! Even so, though I had enough numbers for most purposes, I would have preferred to have had a complete year's records. But that timetable would have upset our own children's school holidays and our annual visit to our parents in

Cape Town. Wife/mother/daughter/doctor roles always needed juggling.

Copying thousands of clinic records of weekly weights in the first year of life needed the same gritting of teeth. But I tend to be tenacious, perhaps obsessive, in finishing any project I've undertaken and find a special gratification in carrying through a worthwhile and decent job.

It is obvious that I cannot summarize the mass of data that I collected—the completed thesis weighs over five pounds! Instead I limit myself to some brief comments on comparative birth weights, growth in the first year of life, and incidence of breast-feeding. In addition I pay some attention to the subject of illegitimate births because of the light it sheds on community mores, family stability, and infant mortality—particularly among Africans.

The advantage of being white in South Africa shows up from birth. At the time of my study the average birth weight of the white babies was 7 lb. 8 oz., a pound heavier than that of the Indian babies. Coloreds at 6 lb. 14 oz. and blacks at 6 lb. 12 oz. occupied an intermediate position between whites and Indians. Conversely, since prematurity is defined on the basis of weight (5 lb. 8 oz. and under), only 4.2 percent of white, but 18.3 percent of Indian babies were classified as premature. Had prematurity been measured in other ways, it is likely that the Indian figure would have been somewhat lower—the average birth weight of Indian babies was only a pound higher than the prematurity standards. Nevertheless, the incidence is very high and the causes of prematurity and low birth weight are the same—largely socioeconomic and cultural—poverty, ill-health of mothers, undernutrition during pregnancy, early childbearing, closely spaced pregnancies, and inadequate prenatal supervision, rather than race per se. We quite commonly found Indian women who weighed less than 100 lb. during pregnancy. In our experience the colored community was the best nourished of the nonwhite groups, followed by the African, and then the Indian.

In comparing growth patterns of the four ethnic groups from two to fifty-two weeks of life, I used all the available records of the Durban Municipal Children's Clinics from 1948–51. As I noted earlier, at the beginning of their lives white babies were the heaviest, Indian babies the lightest, and colored and black babies intermediate between the two. By the end of the year white babies were still the heaviest, but black babies had overtaken the colored infants. Indian babies grew as fast as whites for about two months, but fell away increasingly thereafter. Black babies overtook white ones at about one month, and maintained their lead until they reached thirty weeks of age after which they dropped below them. In interpreting these results, I suggested that white infants were underfed in early life due to strictly regulated, by-the-clock schedules of nursing. Pediatricians at that time lectured mothers on the danger of overfeeding. Babies of the other ethnic groups grew well in early life due to their mothers' accepted practice of nursing on demand. But when the latter's children needed other foods in addition to breast milk, the mothers could neither afford the purchase nor were they sufficiently educated in child nutrition. I was fortunate in having access to records of Durban middle-class babies of all races who used the services of a privately practicing pediatrician. Her charts did not show the characteristic slowing of growth of black, colored, and Indian infants.

South African mothers of all races were way ahead of U.S. mothers in the proportion who breast-fed. At the time of discharge from hospital, between seven and nine days after giving birth, 98.6 percent of black, 97.9 percent of colored, 93.4 percent of white, and 71.1 percent of Indian babies were fed solely on breast milk. Very few of the Indian babies were on the bottle only, but a substantial number supplemented breast milk with cow's milk. We believed that the poor nutritional state of the Indian mothers—due largely to a most inadequate intake of calories and protein—plus their high fertility rates resulting in big families with closely spaced births, was probably responsible for their difficulty in establishing a sufficiency of milk.

Perhaps the most revealing area of my study was the situation regarding illegitimacy in the four groups. As a doctor I was interested in illegitimacy for the effect it had on infant morbidity and mortality, but in searching for the figures and trying to interpret them, I learned a great deal about community mores and the effects of the white dominant culture on the habits of other ethnic groups. There were two groups of Indians in Durban—the "Indian Immigrants"—a mainly Hindu group, descendants of the Indians brought from India from 1860 onward by the government of Natal to work as indentured laborers in the sugar fields or as domestic and general laborers. The "Passenger Indians," on the other hand were free Indians—mainly Moslem—who paid their own passage from India and settled as traders among the indentured Indians. (They were a small group which I did not use in my growth studies.) Passenger Indians had the highest percentage of married mothers, 99.3 percent. Whites followed closely behind with 98.4 percent married, hardly differing from Indian Immigrant mothers with 98.2 percent. Colored figures dropped considerably to 69.9 percent, and blacks fell lower yet—only 47.4 being married.

Strong social disapproval was shown to white unmarried mothers and to their offspring. In almost all such cases these babies were not breast-fed and were put up for adoption. As I indicated, illegitimacy was almost unheard of among Moslem Indians. So strong was family solidarity among them, and so closely were their daughters guarded, that Indian health assistants at the Institute of Family and Community Health expressed surprise that any illegitimacy at all was found in this community. The Hindu community was also very strict in its attitude to premarital conception. The young girls were closely chaperoned and traditional marriage customs were maintained. Caste regulated marriage and, especially among upper-caste families, violation of regulations involved out-casting. Marriage was a family affair, and there was no divorce among the Hindu. The family regarded illegitimate conception as a disgrace and the mother, though not the child, was stigmatized. Hindu girls who became pregnant before marriage have been known to commit suicide rather than bear the disgrace.

The attitude of the colored people of Durban to illegitimacy varied, depending on whether the parents were country folk or town people. Country parents were much stricter and deplored their daughters' "bad ways." In the town illegitimacy had perforce been accepted but with shame. No stigma attached to the child, and the unmarried mother often married subsequently. Studies of the colored community of Durban showed a lack of family cohesion, unifying tradition, and close community life.

Africans presented a different and more severe problem. Here the change of attitude was marked and rapid. Customary marriage had been legalized by transfer to the wife's people of *lobola*—generally in the form of cattle—thus legitimizing the marriage and resultant offspring. Children born to a woman for whom *lobola* had not been paid were regarded as illegitimate and belonged to the mother's family, and a child of an adulterous union belonged to its sociological, not its natural, father. But the *lobola* system changed over time becoming more of a commercial transaction with money taking the place of cattle. There had also been a marked change in the relationship between parents and their children. The decline of ancestor worship deprived the father of his role of family priest, and the abolition or modification of the old initiation ceremonies led to a slackening of family discipline. Labor migration cut off parental authority for long periods of time, and sons also migrated to the towns living independently from their families. With the absence of young men and the decline of polygamy, sexual life in the reserves was affected, and in the towns the large floating population of unattached men led inevitably to casual unions and an increase of prostitution. Under these conditions illegitimacy became common, as reflected in my figures. Parents, while extremely worried about this, could not prevent it from happening.

In Lamontville the percentage of illegitimate births, 28.4 percent, was about half that for Durban as a whole, but the usual problem of under registration of births delivered outside of hospitals made the Durban figure unreliable. The contrast between the accurate black rates—gathered by health center staff—and the equally accurate Indian rates of the Indian health center remained striking, 28.4 percent versus 3.9 percent. In both groups the illegitimate births occurred most often in young mothers. Illegitimacy rates are important, not only as a measure of family and community stability, but also because they correlate positively with infant mortality rates. In a study of infant mortality among three Zulu and two Hindu communities, all served by health centers of our Institute, the highest infant mortality rate recorded, 192.7, was among the black rural people in Polela in the first four years of that center's operation. The lowest rate, 48.2 percent was found among the Hindu population living in the subeconomic housing project of Springfield, again in its center's first four years.[5]

Two doctors, a male surgeon and I, got M.D. degrees in 1955; at this time I was the second woman at the University of Cape Town to get that qualification. The spouse of the first woman was an editor of one of Cape Town's two daily newspapers, and he sent a reporter to interview me. I refused, not wanting the publicity. When the editor himself called, I agreed to be interviewed on condition that he limited the published information to my name and the subject of the thesis. I never even thought about newspaper captions. The paragraph appeared as I had stipulated, but above it was the reason the editor had wanted the interview: "Mother of Four Gets M.D.!"

My own mother, proud of her daughter's achievement as mothers are, insisted that I accept her gift of a ceremonial, red doctorate gown. (I had intended to rent a gown for the graduation.) The gown, resplendent (and expensive), was made by a military tailor, and since Harry would be getting his M.D. a little later, I asked the tailor to make the gown to fit him also. He complied only too well—it fitted Harry better than it did me—and with true male, military chauvinism he stitched Harry's name in it and left mine out! Still, it was fun being allowed to have the children attend the graduation ceremony with Harry, and I took great care not to trip on the stairs in that too long gown.

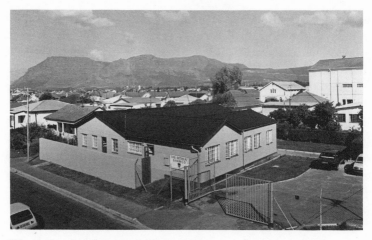

"The Retreat," SHAWCO's *children's home*

In the summer of 1983 we visited family and friends in South Africa. On our second last day in Cape Town, Harry was told by his nephew that he owned a small house on the Cape Flats. Apparently willed to him by his father, it had been rented for a sum so small that it paid only for the taxes. But his nephew had recently renovated the house, paying for this by charging a higher, more reasonable rent. He asked Harry what he wanted done with it. Harry recoiled in horror. He thought he'd taken out whatever had been left to him by his father (who had been dead for thirty years) and wanted no truck with this property. "I don't want it. Sell it," he said. His nephew pointed out that this might be no easy matter. The present tenant was colored, though the surrounding neighbors were white, and there was talk of the area becoming "for whites only" under the Group Areas Act. Harry's distaste was obvious. He refused to go and see the cottage; he wanted no part of it. If there was difficulty in selling it, he would give it away as soon as he'd decided on a suitable recipient.

For several weeks, after we got home, we discussed possible recipients. In the mail, at that crucial time, we got the 1984 UCT alumni magazine telling about SHAWCO's latest accomplishments. The decision was made immediately: Harry wrote to UCT's vice-chancellor and principal offering him the house to be used for the benefit of SHAWCO. UCT sold the house, realizing almost R10,000 for it, and used the money toward furnishing "Retreat," the new Children's Home for abused and neglected children that SHAWCO had recently built.

We heard indirectly that Harry's family thought his gift quixotic to say the least: "It would have paid for two visits to South Africa." But Harry was very pleased with what he had done. In a small way he was repaying a debt.

Emigrating

I note with pride, and some self-shame, that young, vigorous students continue to demonstrate their concerns over inequalities and inequities in South African society. But many young people have left South Africa—as we did—unable any longer to lead the kind of schizophrenic existence of white, privileged people living in a political system where skin color determines position in society. The country's loss is keen and accelerating and in Helen Suzman's words a great indictment of the government.

Some of our colleagues were forced out. Bill Hoffenberg, a friend and distinguished endocrinologist at the University of Cape Town, and married to Margaret, the first SHAWCO director of welfare, was "banned" by the South African Government—no reason given. Though Bill fought strenuously against the banning order, he lost the battle and went to Britain with Margaret in 1967. Fourteen years later Bill was elected president of the Royal College of Physicians of England, was knighted by the Queen, and is now president of an Oxford college. An article in a Cape Town daily newspaper, reporting Bill's election, deplored the "arbitrary 'security' process" by which he was hounded out of South Africa and commented, sadly, on the brain drain resulting from Nationalist actions and policies.

We are grateful that Harry's decision to emigrate was made while our children were still young. He didn't want them to grow up in South Africa. They agree, saying that if we had stayed, they surely would have left sooner or later, and it would have been impossible to remain a close family. Many of our friends who remained now have children in Britain, Canada, the United States, Australia, and Israel. Yet there are still times when I am ambivalent about whether we were right to run away, and I think of that brave resistance fighter, Helen Joseph, who calls leaving the ultimate betrayal.

Our decision to leave was made several years before it happened. When the Nationalist government was elected for the second time in 1952, and with an increased majority, we knew we would go. But where?

As it happened, Harry's father—all of whose siblings had settled in the United States—paid our fares to visit his family, and our round trip tickets to see these U.S. relatives enabled us to explore four countries as possible places to settle in.

Britain was our obvious, first choice. We had grown up on British literature and had absorbed the colonial mythology of absolute British superiority in all things. Our medical teachers had been British or British-trained; we had worked as interns in British hospitals; our degrees would have been recognized, and we liked the prospect of becoming a part of Britain's recently instituted National Health Service. We knew we couldn't become hospital consultants since we weren't trained as specialists, and we wouldn't become general practitioners because we didn't want to set up in practice. But we could be medical officers of health because we each had the necessary public health degree, based on the British model. Optimistically, we discussed this possibility with several people in the health service. To our surprise they warned that after our years in South Africa's innovative health centers we would find the work of British health officers exceedingly dull—and advised against it.

Our second choice, Israel, also presented good and bad sides. We wouldn't be lonely since we had several relatives living there; our medical degrees would be recognized; the country had a strong Labor government, and we were attracted by the ideals of the kibbutz communities. Most importantly, we could contribute to the building up of this old/new country—giving us a positive instead of a negative reason for leaving South Africa. On the other hand living conditions in Israel were extremely tough. The government was chronically short of money; both of us would have to work full-time to earn a pittance, and our knowledge of Hebrew was decidedly meager. Real refugees from Europe and the Middle East needed housing and were being moved from tents to hastily built apartments. At best we might manage to get a two-room apartment. After four-and-a-half years of the army Harry had had his fill of barracks and wanted a different kind of life. Even so we might have overcome these negative reactions if we had been fervent nationalists, but we were internationalists in our philosophy and decided to look elsewhere.

Canada appealed, especially Saskatchewan whose Socialist government had started a model health care program for the province. A new medical school had been built in Saskatoon, and Harry liked the thought of working at this school and being active in the provincial plan. I recall that it was mid-August at the time we visited and that Saskatoon was flat as a pancake, devoid of beauty, hot, and dry. Politely I enquired about the climate, to be told blithely, "There are four months in the year without killing frost." Shuddering in anticipation of the winter, I told Harry I didn't fancy living in Saskatoon, but if we *had* to I wouldn't stand in his way, and I would do my best to adapt. "Perhaps I could acclimatize by starting to put my head in the refrigerator for a few hours every day." Harry, surprised at my unusual opposition, chided me. "It's the political climate, not the meteorological, that counts." "Maybe so," I retorted, "but the meteorological climate certainly helps." To my intense relief Harry didn't get the job.

That left the United States. We, or at least I, hadn't seriously considered America. We couldn't get our medical registration there without writing stiff exams, and some states even demanded a repeat internship. We weren't familiar with the U.S. medical system and didn't know where we'd fit in. In addition, the cost of living was far beyond what we were used to in South Africa. But as we traveled across the continent—there were relatives from New York to San Francisco—we found much warmth and friendliness. At each stopping-off place we met caring colleagues who referred us to others in the town we were due to visit next. We told them we wouldn't feel comfortable in private practice, but many of the doctors we met believed in a national health service for the United States or at least in national health insurance to cover medical costs for all citizens. We learned of new, exciting programs in public health and in community medicine. As we had done in the other three countries, so we did in the U.S.: explained why we wanted to emigrate, noted names and addresses of those who seemed sympathetic, and asked for help in finding suitable jobs.

Meanwhile, in 1954 Harry became Senior Lecturer in Social Medicine at the University of Cape Town. So we returned to live in Cape Town and marked time until we could find work overseas. U.S. immigration regulations required a two-year hiatus between possession of a visitor's visa and the granting of a "green card" entitling aliens to live and work in America.

Unexpectedly, the most attractive, overseas job that came up a couple of years later was in Boston—a city we hadn't visited since we had confined ourselves to cities with relatives. It happened through American generosity and friendliness, because people we had contacted took trouble on our behalf and got in touch with others in different cities whom we hadn't met. A post for Harry as lecturer in the Department of Public Health Practice at the Harvard School of Public Health sounded very attractive, the more so since it would ensure a first priority entry visa—much sought after and not easy to get. The snag was that it offered no security beyond eighteen months when the grant which funded the job would end, and Harry would have to begin work within three months. Having decided to take the job, Harry continued at his old job until the Friday before the Tuesday on which he was to begin his new one. He had to finish writing his M.D. thesis and didn't want to lose a month's salary; plus he needed to find accommodation for the family. It was a clear and expected division of responsibility—his to go ahead and start our new life, mine to stay behind to settle our affairs and then follow with the children.

Harry landed in New York on February 20, 1956. We arrived on April 16, after a hectic eight-weeks interval, which left me little time to brood over the pain of leaving our homeland or the fear of confronting a new world of strangers. In this interim I busied myself editing and proofreading Harry's completed thesis, selling our house and furniture, deciding what we would take with us, and sorting and discarding books and files. We were a "book" family, and I remember telling the children that they could only take with them the books they felt they could not live without. I sold our car to an understanding friend who let me keep it till the day we left. So, in our last week I was able to show our children some of the places I cared about most: the university, the beautiful old Windmill, the protea gardens at Kirstenbosch, the avenue which went through the original vegetable gardens planted by the Dutch East India Company, the winding road around Chapman's Peak overlooking the Atlantic Ocean, the fishing village of Hout Bay where we used to buy crayfish for eighteen pence apiece, and Cape Point, meeting place of the Atlantic and Indian oceans, where David as the oldest male in the family quickly picked up a stick to protect us from the wild baboons we saw sitting on the rocks. I kept the best for the last—an ascent by cable car to the top of Table Mountain to see the city we loved and were about to lose spread below us. The air was so still we could hear a dog barking.

On each such journey I wondered if this would be the last time we would witness these scenes, and I wanted desperately to imprint them on the children's minds. "Look," I would tell them, "look hard and remember." And, except for Philip who was less than two, they remembered much of what they saw.

Now, writing about that last week in South Africa, I can't really explain why it was so important to me that the children be able to recall what they had seen or what difference it could possibly have made to them in the United States whether they remembered or not. Yet, in 1983, when we decided to visit South Africa after a period of work in Swaziland, Mark wanted to come with us. He needed to fill in the gaps in his memory, recover

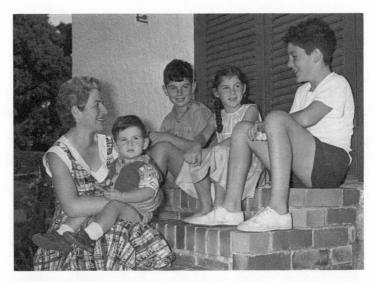

Just before we emigrated

the missing pieces, trace the pattern of his early life. When it was over, he likened the journey to a retrospective exhibition.

The difficulties of leaving included giving away Panda, our beautiful collie—how the children and I hated that! I was heavy-hearted the day our household goods were auctioned off to strangers, our dishes, curtains, rugs, our beautiful indigenous, hardwood living-room furniture—a present from Harry's parents. The children were staying with Bertie and Betsy, Harry's brother and sister-in-law, but I spent the night of the auction alone in the stripped house, sleeping on the floor. I had to be by myself to come to terms with leaving family and friends, our house, our city, our country, which we loved but into which we no longer fitted.

Of course the shock of being uprooted varies markedly with individuals and their circumstances.[1] Harry, in contrast to me, was so anxious to pull out of South Africa that he was excited rather than sad at going, but I left reluctantly, with more sorrow and guilt. If all socially conscious doctors left South Africa, who would do our kind of work?

I hadn't anticipated the extent of the physical burden that traveling alone with four young children would entail—first to Johannesburg and then thirty-eight hours of flying time to New York. However, far worse than that, and completely unexpected, was the behavior of a friend who took the opportunity presented by my journey to time a visit of her very deaf mother to her American brother. I agreed to look after her mother, but insisted that she not request the seat next to me since the airline had assured me I'd have a complete row of five seats for the family— the three on the one side of the aisle and the two on the other side. They would book no one else in our row; Philip, aged twenty-two months, would definitely have a seat. Painfully for us, both friend and airline reneged on their promises. The mother—whose hearing aid malfunctioned as soon as we were aloft—was assigned the seat on my left, Rosalie, age six, sat on my right, Philip's only seat was my lap, and my two older boys of twelve and nine were put in seats in the row behind us.

Philip, normally a happy, talkative child, was accustomed to running around freely and unfettered. Bewildered at the change from his normal routine, missing his home and the loving attention of the adults he was used to, afraid of the strange toilets, having no idea what the journey was all about, he bawled, it seemed, continuously, in misery and protest. One young woman on our plane traveled with a baby of a few months and a three-year-old. Returning to the plane with her older child after a stop in Lisbon, she suddenly discovered that she had left her baby behind in the ladies' restroom and the plane was delayed while she rushed to retrieve her infant. Passengers tut-tutted disapprovingly, but I could appreciate the strain she was under. It was the most wretched journey of my life. Though I recognized that the role of breadwinner was regarded as primarily the husband's and the responsibility for home and children the wife's, on that journey I would happily have reversed the roles.

In New York Harry was waiting to escort us to Boston. My relief was intense, but rest was still several hours away. Harry had been staying at the home of a physician who, thinking the exposure good for his children, occasionally rented rooms to foreigners. Generously, he offered us temporary shelter in the family attic, plus the use of a refrigerator in the basement. I was terrified that Philip might roll down flights of stairs if I was absent for a few minutes and he went in search of me, but that first night I was beyond worrying about the future. I had hardly slept since we left Cape Town and craved sleep so much that for the first time ever I didn't hear my baby crying in the night, though we all shared one big room. Luckily, Rosalie was a very motherly sister, and as I slept through his cries, she woke, gave him his bottle, and soothed him back to sleep. We had arrived in our new land.

I think back, occasionally, to that irksome flight. Life in South Africa (for whites) was so comfortable, so soft, so free of irritants that we weren't inured to hardship. And then I think how lucky I was not to be born two generations earlier. My grandmother had told me, in vivid detail, of her voyage from Lithuania with her two teenage daughters when she came to join her husband in Cape Town. Fleeing pogroms and the appalling harassment of Jews in Czarist Russia, they traveled steerage under wretched conditions for a whole month. They took with them their clothes, their feather beds, their pots and pans. Being orthodox Jews, they couldn't eat nonkosher shipboard food. On that long journey they subsisted on black bread, pickled herrings, and potatoes.[2]

Part Two. Boston

A decent provision for the poor is the true

test of civilization.

—*Samuel Johnson*

Becoming a Housewife

When we came to Boston in 1956, we were surprised how few people we met knew anything about South Africa. To many our country was a vast land populated mainly by wild animals and black people scantily dressed in beads and skins—situated somewhere near Australia. Harry still tells about people at the Harvard School of Public Health who asked whether he'd had much trouble with the Mau Mau, and how he delightedly pointed out that the Mau Mau were as far from Cape Town as the Panama Canal from Boston. But we too were ignorant.

Rosalie told us, recently, that as a child listening to an aunt talking about American television and food habits—South Africa only introduced television in the 1970s with separate channels for whites and blacks—she thought we were going to live in a very funny country. She expected to find lots of people who lived in little boxes and to eat all her food out of cans. Like most immigrants, Harry and I thought in terms of large cities: size, skyscrapers, neon lights, heavy traffic, noise, variety of people. We knew little of small-town rural America, differences in outlook between East and West, North and South. We had never heard of the Bible Belt or realized that the Civil War was as close to Southerners as the Boer War to Afrikaners. Despite the McCarthy period and the still subservient role of the blacks, we were hopeful, because we automatically made comparisons to South Africa—and here we believed that the law was good and the people were free.

Perhaps most strange was our ignorance of the medical care system. We admired the British national health service and knew such a system didn't exist in the States, but we'd met fine

Americans in medical care and, on the basis of these individuals, were optimistic about the direction that medical care would take.

Friends who settled in England, particularly south of London, told us of their difficulty with the aloofness and reserve of the English—those who Jean Rhys describes as people who touch life with gloves on. We never had this problem in Boston—Americans must be among the world's most outgoing, friendly, and hospitable citizens. On the other hand we found many of them surprisingly parochial in outlook, thinking their country superior to all others in every respect. For instance, many Bostonians found it hard to understand that Harry could have been offered a job sight unseen by their country's most famous university. Later, when I too worked at Harvard, and later still when our children went there to college, our story became yet more incomprehensible. Our questioners usually concluded that Harry and I must have been educated in England, for they doubted we could have achieved "American standards" of education in South Africa.

In our early years in Boston we often thought of Churchill's remark that Britain and America were two countries divided by a common language. We had problems understanding others and making ourselves understood—particularly when shopping for essentials. We heard Philip at times repeating common words in the two languages: lorry and truck, wireless and radio, bucket and pail, spade and shovel (I still get mixed up at times). The older children learned a simplified spelling, different pronunciation, new rules in punctuation, the superiority of baseball and basketball to cricket and rugby, and the magnetic power of television. Harry and I learned to drive on the right instead of the left, to shop in supermarkets, to carry our own brown paper grocery bags instead of having our goods delivered, and to live in a do-it-yourself world instead of one made thoughtlessly easy by an abundance of cheap labor. More difficult for all of us was knowing nobody in Boston. We will always remember how, the first time we went to a concert in Boston's Symphony Hall, we looked around at intermission and recognized not one person. In Cape Town on similar occasions we knew half the audience.

It was this early loneliness that over the years contributed to our house becoming a kind of shelter for South African immigrants and visitors to Boston. We gained a lot from these contacts—enjoying the warm companionship of a surrogate extended family, in some instances making lifelong friends. For a while we even kept a South African visitors' book. American guests, listening to South Africans reading aloud the names of previous guests and discussing their present whereabouts, would ask in surprise whether all South Africans knew each other. We South Africans in our diaspora knew we could rely on our compatriots, just as a generation earlier our parents aided each other when they left Russia for a new country.

Once a young woman telephoned for assistance. I listened to the familiar accent spilling out a tale of woe: she was eight months pregnant and needed the name of a good obstetrician; her husband had just begun a radiology residency at the Massachusetts General Hospital; they'd been in the country only ten days and didn't know their way around; they desperately needed a place to stay other than the expensive hotel in which they were temporarily located. I heard her through without interruption before I asked: "Do I know you?" "No," she answered, "but my mother knows your sister."

I knew I could trust anyone my sister steered to me for help. We were due to leave in a few days for a short vacation with Harry's American aunt in Pennsylvania, and it seemed a good idea to shelter the couple in our house while we were gone, leave them a list of real-estate agents, obstetricians, telephone numbers of our good friends, and so on. So we invited them over, showed them around the house, and gave them the spare set of house keys.

When we reported the incident to our aunt, she was horrified.

"How can you leave your house to a perfect stranger?" she exclaimed.

"She's not a stranger," I countered. "Her mother knows my sister."

My family teased me on our way home telling me there'd be a new baby in our house for me to look after, but all was well. The young woman and her husband had found an apartment, she had seen an obstetrician, and we became friends.

Just as those new arrivals were anxious about their future, so were we. Harry had been the mainspring of our move, but could guarantee our financial support for eighteen months only—a worrisome responsibility. The children had been cut off from close relatives and good friends (Mark confided later how much he minded the absence of cousins in Boston), but I think the change was hardest on me, as it would have been on any woman in my position. Husbands meet interesting people at work; children quickly make friends at school; women, particularly those who'd previously had fulfilling jobs, are faced with lonely and constricted lives. Harry had come to a job in Boston, but I didn't know where I'd fit in.

The older children managed well, but they weren't used to the noisiness of the classrooms and the lack of discipline that seemed to be the norm. Rosalie, aged six, her eyes wide with astonishment, reported to me: "Mommy, you should hear the way the children talk to the teacher!" In Mark's class the children had been told that a boy from Africa would be joining them and were most disappointed to find he was just a white boy like all the rest of them. According to the substitute teacher (who later became a friend) Mark, on being asked to describe his home in South Africa, obligingly drew a picture of the house on the blackboard. (I wish I knew what his classmates expected our house to look like—a thatched-roofed hut perhaps?) David had the most exciting introduction to his school. He was asked if he could do a Zulu warrior war dance. Though he'd never witnessed such a dance, David, undaunted, performed in front of an admiring audience, who fortunately, had no better idea than he about who or what a Zulu warrior was or how he danced. We marveled that our boys, painfully shy as they were, could manage with such aplomb. But Philip was desperately unhappy.

I'd done a lot of work with babies, and Philip was our fourth child, yet I hadn't anticipated Philip's distress. The others were old enough to understand, at least in part, the reasons for our move; to Philip at twenty-two months it was incomprehensible. His safe, secure, happy world had been shattered. He was bewildered, and he grieved. Luckily, he was an early talker which helped us understand what he was going through. Each day for several months he repeated the names of those adults who'd lived in his home but were no longer with him—his granny, Katy his nanny, Sakkie.

Though he ordinarily drank from a cup, I gave him bottles in the airplane thinking it might prevent earache. He also had his pacifier. When we finally settled down in a permanent home, Philip and I had long, daily discussions on why he should discard first the bottle and then the pacifier. He understood the message intellectually, would nod his head in assent, and say "tomorrow." And he wouldn't let me out of his sight. If others could disappear, so could I.

After some months of having Philip constantly with me, I tried nursery school. As long as I sat there he was fine. When I got up to go, he panicked. Eventually I called a very sensible child psychiatrist for advice. "Are you sure," he asked, "that he can't bear to have you leave? Or is it that you can't bear to leave him?" I conceded, left Philip to cry at nursery school, and he quickly settled down. But for a long time I remained overanxious. I had never forgotten that Mark, at about Philip's age, had barely escaped the wheels of a truck when he ran across the road after spotting me parking opposite his nursery school. When Philip was old enough to ride his first tricycle up and down the two sidewalks of our corner house, I ran from window to window inside the house following his progress and making sure he wouldn't wander into the street. I didn't understand why, in cities with their surprisingly meager child-care facilities and their horrendous traffic, it was considered unneighborly, un-American, to build a wall or fence around one's house.

Petty differences in child-rearing between our two countries I simply ignored. The daughter of our American aunt, visiting us soon after we arrived, took me aside to point out the error of my ways with Philip. "Only very poor children of uneducated parents walk around without shoes and pee (I'm not sure what word *she* used) in the garden." I made a mental note to be more discreet on her next visit.

Our first three weeks of living in an attic were hard on all of us, though I tried to hide my nostalgia, my unsettled feeling, my anxiety, and my sense of isolation. Yet now when I think back to those days, I can see that the very stringency of our situation forced me to be resilient and adapt quickly. On our second or third day in Boston, Harry dropped the children off at school on his way to work. I was to walk them home accompanied by Philip. But that day, past mid-April, it snowed. None of us had suitable winter coats, hats, and shoes, and a stroller was hardly snowproof. Not quite desperate enough to call Harry at work, I learned about the yellow pages and arranged for the children to be brought home by cab. I couldn't leave Philip alone at home: four steep flights of ungated stairs joined attic and basement.

After those three weeks, during which I tried out a large variety of American canned food that could be heated on a hot plate placed on a board over the bathtub—confirming Rosalie's belief—we moved into the house Harry had rented in Brookline. We bought a television while we lived there to stop the children spending their after-school hours glued to a neighbor's set. This house was tucked away on a steep side street within easy walking distance of a busy thoroughfare. It was a pleasant dwelling with a small front yard and a rather deep drop to a tangle of vegetation at the back. Fully furnished, it also contained a large collection of bric-a-brac, some of which was kept in glass-fronted cabinets. Dr. Hawes, a Presbyterian minister and the owner, explained that he would not have rented his home to an American family with children, but since we were "British" our children could be trusted not to break his china. When we moved into our own house Philip used to look at objects and ask: "Can I touch? Is this ours or Dr. Hawes's?"

While Harry worried about our financial future, I was concerned about the care of the children and the running of the house. Unfortunately, I was woefully ill-prepared for housewifery: in those early months there were many times I would gladly have traded my professional skills for skills in housekeeping.

Strangely, during an unusually heavy snowfall in Chapel Hill, I dreamed about our first winter in Boston and woke laughing ruefully. I was dressing Philip in his snowsuit and boots to take him to nursery school, and, as usual, it triggered his immediate need to go to the bathroom. Meanwhile Rosalie—afraid she'd be late for school—clamored to get her hair braided. (I had a love/hate relationship with her silky, dark-brown, beautiful tresses—so long she could almost sit on them—which I could never plait as tightly as Katy had done. When Rosalie went to college she cut her hair, but on a recent visit she turned to me and with a smiling face but a remorseful voice asked, "Mom, how could you let me do it?")

But, no matter my deficiencies, I tried to follow ridiculous South African standards of house cleaning. It was the custom there to polish floors and wash windows very frequently—weekly it seems to me, but I could be exaggerating. Shirts, sheets, and towels were ironed, and I had witnessed many a Madam finger-testing for dust. After I had exhausted myself with such madness the first few weeks, I relaxed my standards—and Harry bought drip-dry shirts. (I had never used a washing machine: in South Africa a washerwoman came to the house on Mondays to do the week's wash, using a scrub board and tub, hung the washing on an outside line, and came back on Tuesdays to iron.) Dr. Hawes had left us an ancient tank-type vacuum cleaner. After Harry left for work and the older children for school, I settled down to clean house. The first time I used the vacuum cleaner, I could hardly wait for David, then aged twelve, to come home from school to tell him about the peculiar behavior of the cleaner, which blew dust out instead of sucking it in. David

listened intently, his face sympathetic, then half-smiled and commented: "You obviously connected the tubes wrongly, Mom; I'll
fix it for you." Relieved at his simple solution, I gave him a bear
hug and went back to cleaning.

I was deeply ashamed that I didn't know how to cook for my
family. Though I never cooked a chicken with the insides left
in, I did equally foolish things. When we left South Africa a
relative gave me an American cookbook—The Woman's Home
Companion—a weighty volume. At the time I debated whether
the knowledge it held could be worth its extra weight, but I took
it with me, and I read it every night for three months. It was
my source of culinary wisdom, my guide and textbook, my equivalent of a child's cuddle-comforter. (Years later, when I no longer
used the book and allowed myself to discard it, I felt grown-up
and triumphant.)

Each day when the cleaning was done, I took Philip in his
stroller to Brookline Village to buy the ingredients which "the
book" decreed I needed for that night's supper. The shopkeepers
began to recognize me, among them Harry of Harry's Fish
Shop—a kindly, grandfatherly man. Whenever I bought fish,
Harry would present Philip with a packet of potato chips. On
the days I didn't buy fish, he'd watch to see when I went by,
dash out of his shop, and give Philip the customary package.
Each day Philip would ask whether we were going to "Harry
the Fish-Shop." I became embarrassed by this generosity and
began to walk on the other side of the street, but Harry would
cross the road with his gift. He'd advise me on which fish was
better fried, broiled, or baked, and one Friday told me he had
just the right fish for me to make "gefilte" fish. My grandmother,
my mother, and Sakkie all made gefilte fish on Fridays, but I
never had. Harry was shocked at my ignorance and offered me
his wife's recipe.

We had been used to having people for meals in South Africa,
a pleasant way to entertain, particularly since I had done very
little of the work. After two or three weeks in Dr. Hawes's house,
we invited our first supper guests, a visiting Scottish nurse and

our young cousin, Peggy, a student at Radcliffe. With some trepidation I decided to make fillets of sole stuffed with shrimp as the main course, and followed directions to the letter. But the book couldn't replace experience in judging when the fish was ready, and I called for help. Our guests taught me common-sense ways of judging readiness, and after supper, seeing how tired I was, insisted I lie down on the couch to rest while they washed the dishes.

After cooking a different meal each night for three months, I recognized with great relief that American cookbooks were written for people like me. Exact amounts of each ingredient were specified, the method of putting the recipe together clearly explained; anyone who could read could cook, and with a little imagination and accumulated experience it wasn't difficult to cook reasonably well. As time went on I bought more cookbooks as a fun way to compensate for my early ignorance. By now I have well over a hundred of them, most of which I use solely for nighttime relaxation reading. I never again attempted a constant change of menus—Harry claims that the family has never since eaten as well!

Eating decent meals was not, however, our major preoccupation. All the time we lived in the Hawes house, we worried about where we'd stay next. Since Harry's contract was guaranteed for such a short while, he felt we should go on living in rented houses until we were properly settled. To me the idea of moving again, when Dr. Hawes came back from his summer home in Maine, to another rented house and perhaps to yet another, was appalling. I wanted us to buy a house, to settle the children, to have our own home. Rightly concerned, Harry countered: "What if we have to move to another city for my next job?" I answered more blithely than I felt, "Then we'll sell the house. The children don't need to worry about moving till it happens." Looking back, I realize how rash I was and how badly it might have turned out, but we were young and buying a house wasn't as bold a move as leaving a country.

Harry gave in, and we began to search for a more permanent home. At this time he had his first taste of American-type,

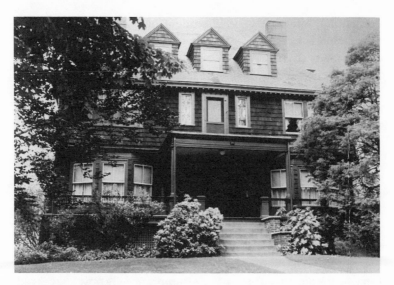

Our Newton home

middle-class, anti-Semitism. He discussed the housing situation with people at work and was taken aback when a very nice secretary advised him not to look for a house in Newton: "Too many Jews there." It's always difficult to know how to react to such remarks, but Harry took them in his stride. "All the more reason to look there, then, since I'm Jewish myself."

One lovely Saturday morning in mid-summer, a real-estate agent took us to see a house in Newton. That house captivated me from the start. It was everything I wanted. When built in 1891, a fine copper-beech had been planted on the front lawn and now majestically shaded that area. Grounds were small, but an apple tree flourished in the backyard, and lilac trees lined the side. Across the street houses bordered a small lake. A spacious house, with beautiful woodwork and several fireplaces, it had a big attic, a huge basement, adequate bedrooms and living-rooms, and a large hall with a handsome, carved staircase leading to the second floor. Though the kitchen and bathrooms were old-fashioned, a lofty shelved pantry adjoining the kitchen delighted me. Shingles on the roof and exterior walls and wooden gutters would soon need replacement, and the porch needed attention. We could also expect trouble with plumbing and wiring, but the house was solidly built and well cared for. Mr. Melcher, the owner, a man in his eighties, had recently been widowed and was leaving his home to live with a married daughter. He confided that no strangers had ever lived in his house, which was built by his wife's parents. His price was $25,000, reasonable enough but $5000 more than the limit we had set ourselves. A mortgage loan required down payment of a quarter of the purchase price, and we had severe monetary constraints.

In 1956 the South African government imposed stringent controls on money leaving the country. A distant connection of mine, with access to "high-ups" in the government, offered to intervene on our behalf to increase our family allowance, but because I couldn't bring myself to accept his offer, we were severely limited in what we could afford for a down payment. We needed, also, to spend money on appliances and furniture.

In our search for another country we had visited the United States briefly but had hardly seen the inside of a house. Almost all who entertained us took us to meals in restaurants—usually ordering huge steaks. Harry's sister, who twice had spent time in the United States, misled us badly about American family life. Most Americans lived in small apartments, she said, used bridge tables for dining, and ate out most of the time or used packaged food. Our furniture, suitable for our big South African house, wouldn't fit into the small apartment in which we would likely live. We knew too little to question her reports. Foolishly, we sold our furniture, on which, unlike cash, there was no export restriction, and in the long run we deprived ourselves of the sense of continuity and comfort that comes from living among familiar possessions.

Despondent, we explained why we couldn't buy the house. Our disappointment was obvious. As we were leaving, Mr. Melcher stopped us and addressed himself to me:

"You really like the house, don't you?"

"Oh, yes!"

"You would take good care of it?"

"Indeed, I would."

"I'll take $20,500."

At that moment I had a flashback to the day when prospective buyers of our last South African home walked through it and, ignoring us, loudly discussed the drastic changes they would make. I remembered our feelings of dismay, and how Harry and I had looked at each other in silent agreement. We would not sell our precious home to *them*. We understood Mr. Melcher's feelings perfectly. After we bought the house, he visited us frequently. Each time he asked me: "Do you still love the house?" I loved it better than any house we lived in, before or since, and grieved to part with it when, fourteen years later, we left Newton for Chapel Hill.

We asked Mr. Melcher to sell us any furniture he didn't want to take with him. Once in a long while I take out his itemized list and marvel, again, at the low prices he charged. Among the two bureaus, mirror, garden tools, carpet sweeper, three beds and mattresses, two bookcases, eight chairs, one side-board, four tables, a step ladder, lawn mower, pair of curtains, fuel oil, fireplace wood and coal, shelving wood, and other miscellaneous items are six small rugs for one dollar each and one larger rug for $15. Entire cost of this miscellany totaled $441.96. We still own the bureaus, a few of the chairs, and three of the rugs. Though we particularly liked those three rugs, we had no idea of their worth until, one day in Chapel Hill, we were visited by an American Indian student whose eyes lit up on seeing the rugs. They were antique Navajo and valuable. Our dog had been sick over one (my washing didn't remove the stain), but the other two I immediately took off the floor and hung on the walls. I like to believe that dear Mr. Melcher must surely have known their true value.

Neighbors were also generous, donating old curtains, a discarded door, odds and ends. Other immediate needs were readily satisfied when we discovered the Salvation Army-type stores and, most of all, Filene's wonderful basement. For years that basement was my treasure trove, supplying clothes for the family, dishes, glasses, pots and pans, and countless other items. I once took a visiting sister-in-law on a journey through the entire store. We began in the basement where she gaped, unbelievingly, at women in our midst trying on dresses without benefit of cubicles. Ascending, we stopped briefly on each floor until we reached the last one—the seventh. There on couches sat expensively garbed women, being waited on by obsequious salesladies bringing out designer clothes one by one. In an hour we had glimpsed all levels of Boston's female society.

Some time after we'd settled in our own home, I began to think—with reservations—about working again professionally. My South African experience had convinced me that, no matter the difficulties, I wanted to go on being a doctor. But I doubted my ability to find and carry a job in this new country. Nobody here knew my previous work; hardly anybody knew I was a doctor; those who did know assumed my name to be Dr. Phillips—the same as my husband's. (After marrying, we intended to change my professional name, but found the cost equal to several months of house-officer salary. By the time we could afford the change, I'd acquired my own professional identity as Salber. It would have been too cumbersome to alter my certificates and explain that letters of reference really belonged to me under another name. Later, holding jobs under my maiden name gave me unearned credit with young women who regarded me as an early, affirmative feminist. Our daughter, who is one, kept her name even on her marriage certificate.)

I had no license to practice, or, for that matter, to drive a car. I had four children, little household help, uncertainty about my competence as a housewife, and memories of deep conflicts between my feelings of responsibility for my family and duty toward the people I'd undertaken to serve. Of all my doubts and fears the easiest to overcome was uncertainty about household competency. I decided to set myself two big tests. Our neighbors in Newton and Harry's colleagues at the School of

Public Health had been extremely kind to us. We invited them to a buffet dinner—all fifty of them. For days I cooked curry; it kept well in our and neighborhood refrigerators, and nobody seemed to mind eating off paper plates. The first test accomplished, the next soon followed. We'd been to dinner at the home of a former British couple in Cambridge, Massachusetts. Her house was the neatest I'd ever seen: not a thing out of place, not a picture askew, not a cushion unplumped. True, she didn't work outside the home, had only one daughter who was in college, and lived in a much smaller house than ours. Nevertheless, she didn't even have a once-a-week charlady—a service I had recently allowed myself. During that visit she recounted tales of spoilt South African women she'd met in Israel during the five years she and her husband had lived there. According to her, some South African women took their colored maids with them to Israel and still needed additional help when they entertained.

I cringed in the collective guilt of privilege and insensitivity of South African housewives and dreaded inviting the couple back. How would I pass inspection? I knew the wife would want to see our house—attic, basement, and all. Gritting my teeth, I set a date for their visit. The charlady and I polished furniture and floors, washed windows and shoved children's toys out of sight in closets. While Harry entertained the husband, I took the wife on a guided tour of the house, which, as I'd anticipated, included attic and basement. At the end she asked: "How do you keep this big house so neat?" I shrugged it off as if it were a mere nothing. South African womanhood had been vindicated, and I had passed my tests.

Soon after I got my Massachusetts driver's license. The hurdles that remained were finding someone I could trust to look after Philip and finding a part-time job. Once more I thought about a live-in nanny—this time a nanny/housekeeper—and decided to aim for the best possible: a Scottish nanny. Letters were dispatched to British agencies. Almost immediately, a seemingly suitable Glaswegian lady offered her services, and we arranged to bring her out. At the last moment she was unable to come, but wrote that a good friend of hers was anxious to take her place. In this way Jean entered our lives and, like Katy, never wanted to leave us. Harry said, later, that just as we had to leave South Africa to free ourselves of Katy, so we had to leave Boston to free ourselves of Jean!

Jean, we discovered, had never been a nanny or a housekeeper. Widowed for many years, she had one child, a married son in his twenties. Most of her adult life had been spent as a worker in a carpet factory; she knew much more about making carpets than housekeeping for a large family. A plain, unimaginative, British-style cook, Jean made excellent fried fish and chips and very good scones. For me, her attractions lay in her soft-spoken manner (her brogue was a delight), her good nature, and most of all her love for Philip, who, in her eyes—and mine—could do no wrong.

Jean blossomed in America, joining three Scottish social organizations as well as the Presbyterian church whose choir she enriched. She went out at night far more than we did, had her meals with us as a family, and relished her new life. We employed her far longer than we really needed her, ensuring that she worked long enough to qualify for U.S. social security abroad. She told us when we visited her later in Glasgow that she should never have left the States, for life had been much better for her there, and she had in Philip the grandson she'd always wanted.

Jean's presence freed me to work if I could find the right job, in actuality a process easier than I'd anticipated. A neighbor we met turned out to be a pediatrician at Children's Hospital in Boston and spoke to a colleague on my behalf. This colleague invited me to join his team of preceptors in his teaching program for Harvard medical students during their rotation through his well-baby clinics. I could supervise as many or as few sessions as I wished. It seemed an opportunity designed specifically to meet my needs.

Before accepting the offer, I discussed the subject at some length with the family. Harry foresaw no problems. David was ambivalent: proud to tell his teacher that his mother as well as his father was a doctor, but thinking Philip still too young for me to be working. Mark was completely supportive. Rosalie wanted me (instead of Jean) to be home when she returned from school each day—confiding later that she would have liked to find me in the kitchen baking cookies as her friends' mothers did. But with three brothers, and an independent nature, she'd always fought for her rights, and she decided I should go back to work. I didn't ask Philip, perhaps because I knew what he would say.

In the end I accepted the work offer on a part-time basis, but I was truly scared to start working in Boston. I took the job because the well-baby field was the one area I was sure I knew more about than did medical students, even those attending the most prestigious medical school in America.

Settling Down at Harvard

My first few sessions of supervising Harvard medical students at well-baby clinics made me wonder if I'd become a reverse racist and a snob to boot. It took some months before I warmed to the predominantly pale-faced babies and to their mothers who arrived at the clinic with curlers in their hair and baby bottles in their hands. (I never got used to the curlers.) The problem, of course, was in me. I missed the African babies, each in its nest on its mother's back or sucking contentedly at her ample breast. How could I expect the Boston babies to smile and gurgle at me if I didn't smile and gurgle first?

My job was to teach medical students how to assess a baby's health: what questions to ask the mother, how to examine the baby, what advice to give until the baby would next be seen. While I could teach students how to take a history and do a thorough examination, when to immunize, and so on, I knew almost nothing about the culture of poor Boston urban mothers who brought their babies to public clinics. Nor did I know what these students had been taught about well babies.

I soon learned that Harvard medical students, who knew a lot about artificial feeding, had been taught almost nothing about breast-feeding, and because doctors and future doctors promoted the product they knew, their advice contributed to the generally low rate of breast-feeding. Mothers who were poor, especially poor black mothers, hardly breast-fed at all. For me, these facts were both a culture shock and an enigma.

Ignorance about breast-feeding wasn't confined to medical students. Later, when I worked in the schools of the Boston suburb where we lived, I talked about nutrition to high school girls taking home economics. At the beginning of the session, I asked them to name the preferred food for very young infants.

"Formula," they replied in one voice.

"What is formula?" My question was followed by some moments of silence.

"I think it's cow's milk," a soft voice ventured.

"Is there any other milk one can give babies?" I asked.

This time there was a long pause before a hand was raised, and a timid voice replied hesitatingly: "I think sometimes goat's milk is used." It looked as if baby bottles would reign for another generation of mothers.

The clinic provided other shocks. There, I first saw disposable syringes, needles, and gloves. In South Africa we had boiled our sparse supply of equipment over and over again. Puzzled, I questioned staff. Because of labor costs, they told me, it was cheaper to throw away material after one use than to spend the time and labor needed for repeated use. But what is discarded by one person is often taken by another; drug addicts regularly searched hospital and clinic bins. Before we threw away our disposable syringes, we broke off their needles to prevent reuse and misuse.

After I'd been working at the clinics for a short while, I was recommended for a research position at the Harvard School of Public Health in the Maternal and Child Health Department. The job as described to me sounded intriguing though vague. For some years staff in that department had served and done research on a mix of poor women and wives of Harvard students during pregnancy and infant rearing. The clinic, now closed, had collected a huge amount of data, filed in numerous, heavy, black volumes which from then on I thought of as the "black books." Dr. Martha Eliot, an elderly, highly respected but somewhat formidable pediatrician, chairman of the department and previously chief of the U.S. government's Children's Bureau, wanted the data analyzed. I was to go through the black books and tell her what research I'd like to undertake. Since I was so puzzled at the low level of breast-feeding in the mothers I'd seen earlier at the clinics, I chose to look at breast-feeding patterns.

Dr. Eliot agreed and allowed me to work half-time as a fellow in maternal and child health. But, because I was not a pediatrician (the fact that I had three medical degrees seemed not to count), my salary would be lowered accordingly. One did not argue with Dr. Eliot.

For the next year or so I labored on those black books. Even in this unusual clinic about 40 percent of the mothers didn't attempt to breast-feed; almost all made this decision during pregnancy. Mothers who'd attended college, particularly those who married men with college education, were the most likely to nurse their babies, but even they weaned their babies very early. The higher the social class of the mother, the more likely she was to nurse. Yet more than half of the mothers of the highest social class nursed their infants for less than three months. The facts were even more startling in women of the lowest social class; over half their babies were weaned by the age of one month. Many reasons were given for rejecting nursing, but an emotional barrier to suckling was the most common. Statements like "I am not a cow" clearly showed embarrassment, even disgust, at the thought of nursing.[1]

I was particularly struck by these results because of the contrast with the behavior of mothers in South Africa. During 1951–52 I studied breast-feeding in Durban, at a time when women remained in hospital for about ten days following childbirth. During that year of study, only one African baby out of 1,482 was bottle-fed when discharged from hospital! In that case the mother had an infected breast, and the baby was fed on the expressed milk of other mothers. The picture was similar for white, colored, and Indian babies. Ninety-six percent of white babies delivered that year at Durban's large provincial hospital went home on mothers' milk.

I knew I couldn't generalize from the Boston clinic results to all Boston mothers. Numbers were small, and the clinic had a disproportionate number of college-educated women who raised the level of nursing. But, later, in 1963, I studied the incidence of breast-feeding among *all* (more than 2,000) babies born in August and September in Boston and two neighboring towns and questioned their mothers by mail and telephone. The contrast with Durban mothers sharpened. Only one-fifth of all these Boston mothers had attempted nursing, and only 5 percent breast-fed their infants for six months or longer. College education and social class had the same positive effect on nursing that I had noted previously. (Ironically, in the twenty-some years since this study, breast-feeding in higher social classes and well-educated mothers has gone on increasing while in the Third World—because of aggressive, commercial promotion of artificial milk—there has been a steady and serious decline.)

Another striking contrast between the United States and South Africa was the difference in poverty levels of the two countries. In our Durban health center, where additional food was often our most effective medicine, we routinely examined every child for signs of malnutrition. Most black children, when they needed solid food in addition to mother's milk, showed the early signs of malnutrition; in weanlings the signs were often gross. In Boston I did the same careful nutritional examinations. Some children were underweight, but not once in the clinics I attended did I find the telltale signs of malnutrition in eyes, mouth, and skin. Poverty in America—at least in Boston—would be riches in Africa.

Memory connects events widely divided in time. On our visit to find another home, in 1953, we had visited Israel and Britain en route to the United States. At that time Britain was still rationing certain foods, and in Israel rationing applied to all foods and was severe. There our diet was mainly sheep-milk cheese and porridge. But in the United States restaurant portions were oversized and often only partly eaten. We would watch with distaste while waiters scooped up leftover food, unused pats of butter, and cigarette ends, which they mixed together and discarded into plastic containers. Watching this, a scene I had long repressed would reappear in my mind's eye. During the year I studied public health in Cape Town, my classmates and I had been taken to inspect the abattoirs. The scene I unwillingly recalled was of large bins filled with gruesome meat condemned by sanitary inspectors as unfit for human consumption. My stomach turned as I remembered being told that in the interval between discarding the meat and its later disposal much of it was regularly stolen by abattoir employees to feed their families. I kept thinking of these marked differences between our old and our new country—universal breast-feeding in the one, bottle-feeding in the other; hunger in the one, waste in the other.

Fortunately for me, the work I did for Dr. Eliot was published, and she was pleased. When my fellowship ended, she offered me another job—exploring areas of research which I thought her department might work on in the future. Her project sounded promising, but the salary she offered was impossible to accept. Because her department was short of cash, Dr. Eliot proposed that I accept a half-time position, be paid for a quarter-time post and think about the job full-time! Such was her power and the awe in which I held her that I tried not to show my negative reaction but asked for time to think about her offer. Arriving home in a turmoil, I turned to Harry for help in finding a good excuse for not taking the job—without offending Dr. Eliot.

Harry had the solution. He'd already written and passed the Massachusetts State Board examination in order to get a medical license. We'd agreed that it would take extraordinary circumstances to make us enter private clinical practice; all the same Harry was sure that our best insurance for the future was for each of us to have a state license. Dr. Eliot would surely understand this argument. She did. For the next two months I studied diligently for the board exams by reading a book written specifically for this purpose. Our six years of medical study, from physics to psychiatry, was crammed into the pages of this book. But medical guilds don't accept foreign medical graduates lightly; they make it difficult even to gain entry to their exams.

It wasn't enough to produce a medical diploma and transcripts of courses taken to get that degree; high-school transcripts were also needed before permission was given to write the exam. (Refugees whose high-school papers were irretrievably lost never could get their Massachusetts licensure.) My high school sent the necessary documents, and after enduring three and one-half days of exams, I passed. If I had failed, I am not at all sure I would have repeated that ordeal.

During the eighteen months I spent as a fellow in maternal and child health, I realized that our South African public health course, based on the British curriculum and designed for training medical officers of health, was of little relevance to the American scene. If I were to remain, as I wished, in the field of public health, it might be wise to enroll in the Harvard School of Public Health for the Master of Public Health degree. Getting that degree seemed to me far better than a medical license as insurance for the future. I applied to be a student, was accepted, and found that we couldn't afford the tuition fees—it made no difference that Harry was on the faculty. As a noncitizen I wasn't eligible for a scholarship; besides, said one committee member, I should be enrolling in the doctoral program, not the masters. However, luck was with me.

Dr. Brian MacMahon, an English physician and chairman of the Department of Epidemiology, knew the British journal where I had published my first few papers on South African infant growth. And, unlike almost all the people I'd met, he knew both my professional name and my previous work. When he offered me a job in his department at the School of Public Health I was too flattered to refuse though I had no academic training in epidemiology. The research I'd done in South Africa, which I thought of as "social medicine," was equated with epidemiology in the United States. When I realized the nature and scope of epidemiology—the basic diagnostic tool for assessing the health and sickness of communities—I became eager to learn its methodology. I began on a part-time basis so I could be readily available to the family, but I found it difficult to limit work hours against the demands of the job. After two years of part-time pay for more than full-time work, I became officially full-time, and I remained in this department for nine years.

For my first epidemiologic research project I chose to survey the smoking behavior of schoolchildren in Newton, Massachusetts. To me, it made much more sense to find out when smoking began, who smoked and why, and then to use this knowledge to educate young people not to start this highly addictive habit than to persuade adults to go through the pain of giving it up. I knew that pain. Though I stopped smoking—"cold turkey"—in 1956 when the first, early reports trickled in, it took a full year before I completely lost all craving for a cigarette. So I designed my study to find out how many boys and girls smoked, at what ages they began to do so, why they smoked, who influenced them, how smokers and nonsmokers differed from each other in social class, achievement at school, personality, and so on. (Looking back I realize that personal reasons of which I was only half conscious at the time also influenced my choice of research topics. Certainly my earlier research in breast-feeding and in comparative growth of white, black, colored, and Indian babies was connected to the current age of our children. At the time of my study on smoking two of our children were old enough to take part in it, and Harry was serving as medical director of Newton's health department.)

During the course of this study, I was excited to learn that a handful of people in other countries were doing the same research I was, and a few articles by these investigators began to show up in the medical journals. But when I started my survey there was no published literature to guide me. Before I plunged into the study itself—I thought I'd use the three high-school classes (grades ten, eleven, and twelve) as my sample—I wanted a population as similar as possible for testing my questionnaire. Among other issues I wanted to test with that class of twelfth graders was whether students would be prepared to sign their papers, for if they would, I could get valuable information impossible without those names. For example, with their names I could link smoking behavior to academic achievement, interview students and their parents, and associate parental smoking with children's smoking. And I could do a follow-up study five years later to see how closely students' anticipation of their own future smoking habits coincided with their actual smoking habits at that time.

But I didn't want the students to tell their friends the questions they were asked and so contaminate the main study. My solution was to use a class of Newton twelfth graders on their last formal day of classes before graduation.

The forty minutes I sat in class waiting to collect the finished questionnaires were forty miserable minutes, for I believed I'd failed badly in my choice of class and day. The unruly students threw paper darts around and generally showed their relief at having finished with school. I expected to find sarcastic, if not downright rude, remarks scribbled on their papers. Instead I found the students had been open, honest, and amenable: almost without exception they signed their names. And several students as they handed me their papers told me that, if I wanted to get a true picture of smoking, I must include the junior high schools in my study. I took their advice: who would know more about the topic? As a result I had almost 7000 students to deal with, seven schools, and dozens of classrooms—all in a very brief space of time. Although this raised horrendous logistical problems, the results more than justified the efforts.

I won't discuss the details of the study nor its results—except for two. In Newton, as opposed to the places where the other investigators worked, I found an unanticipated amount of smoking in girls. More boys than girls smoked in the seventh to the tenth grades, but by the eleventh grade there was no difference between them, and more girls than boys smoked in the twelfth grade.[2] In addition, I found a high level of smoking among Newton mothers.[3] These results were a portent of a larger trend in the nation itself—lung cancer has now overtaken breast cancer as the most important cancer in American women.

An unexpected side effect of the smoking study was the publicity I got. I was becoming better known under my professional name, but my friends knew me as Phillips, which sometimes led to amusing incidents. The study would be discussed in my presence without awareness of my role in it. A friend, who knew the work I was doing, called me indignantly to tell me that she'd read a newspaper report which credited someone called Salber for my work!

It was fun to be sought after by the media and to be invited to national and even international meetings. When I was asked to be a member of a panel to discuss techniques and evaluation of antismoking campaigns, at an international cancer conference in Tokyo, I could hardly believe my luck.

The conference was planned a year in advance, plenty of time to prepare a paper and to read about the wonders of Japan. Chartered flights had been arranged and fares were so reasonable that Harry agreed to attend the meeting with me and to take an additional week of vacation for travel after the conference. He was sent the "spouse program" detailing visits to scenic sites, silk factories, pearl-divers, and so on. Obviously, spouses at professional meetings were (are?) thought of as women only. Harry had little interest in silks and pearls and attended the lectures, but I confess that at times my own mind wandered from viruses to Shinto shrines, kabuki, and wood-block prints.

I was beginning to organize my next project (while continuing to write reports based on analyses of the smoking data) when one of the national television networks decided to produce a documentary on the collision of interest between persons who grew and manufactured tobacco and those whose health could be affected by use of their products. The network wanted me to do a fair amount of work for them, but I was busy and kept on refusing. Eventually, I agreed that cameramen could film a presentation I'd already promised the high school, in which I was including a panel of schoolchildren. It was then I realized fully the astonishing power of television. Parents of panel children were delighted; the school virtually closed down on the morning of the presentation. And, finally, I agreed to one interview in the New York television studio.

Wearing a new shocking-pink dress I'd bought for the occasion, I flew to New York, took a cab to the studio, and met the chief cameraman. He took one quick and disapproving look at me in that new dress.

"Wrong color!" he proclaimed.

Duly chastened, but unable to do anything about the offending dress, I answered the four or five questions that Harry Reasoner asked me, and took the first flight back to Boston. Having learned what color *would* have been right for television I didn't get the opportunity to practice my newly acquired wisdom, for never again did I do work that appealed to a national network.

However, interest in topics seems to be cyclical. I'd considered the Newton study forgotten when it was no longer cited in bibliographies of younger investigators. But apparently it still had a place. Recently, I was called by a young woman investigator in a newly formed Institute for the Study of Smoking Behavior and Policy, at the John F. Kennedy School of Government. She wanted to work on the "natural history of smoking" and hoped to interview, at their twenty-fifth reunion, the twelfth grade class I'd questioned. Would I give her access to their files? I'd promised confidentiality and could not, but, if pressed, I could have written to these alumni and asked their permission. Meanwhile, I referred her to Dr. MacMahon to find out whether the files still existed. They'd been shredded only a few years earlier to make room for new material. (How can one possibly know what data to keep and for how long?)

For several years I was involved in another epidemiologic study, where the people and the venue were distinctly different. I've written earlier about my interest in breast-feeding. Not only did I believe breast milk to be the best food for babies, but in South Africa, where 100 percent of black mothers breast-fed their infants for prolonged periods, we never saw a black mother with breast cancer. I was convinced that breast-feeding protected these mothers from developing breast cancer and wanted to study this as my next research subject. But Dr. MacMahon had already investigated this supposed protective effect in New York—with negative results. I argued that few American mothers breast-fed their infants and those who did hampered lactation by their strict attention to nursing by the clock and by their very early introduction of solid foods to the babies' diets—in vogue at the time.[4] I looked for a population of U.S. mothers who breast-fed amply, whom I could follow and compare with women who didn't breast-feed, and learned of a milk bank that had existed at the Boston Lying In (later the Boston Hospital for Women). Sadly these records had also been shredded. However, Dr. MacMahon saw enough merit in my reasoning to plan a project that would settle the controversy decisively.

Accordingly, he designed and directed an international seven-country study—the countries selected on the basis of having high, intermediate, and low rates of breast cancer. I was put in charge of the American center which (after preliminary work on my part) we designated as Boston and its eight suburbs south of the Charles river. Each center used the same questions in interviewing hospitalized women with breast cancer to test the hypothesis that prolonged lactation protects women against developing cancer of the breast.

Twenty-seven hospitals and many hundreds of doctors in this Boston region treated breast cancer patients. Some of these hospitals saw only a few women with the illness; the Harvard teaching-hospitals, predominantly the Massachusetts General, saw the most and were the most prestigious. If I couldn't persuade the Mass. General to come into the study, we couldn't proceed, for that hospital handled about half of all the cases—without them we couldn't get the magic 80 percent response rate that science (and our chairman) demanded for validity. But, if the Mass. General did agree, I could then approach, and probably get the consent of, the Peter Bent Brigham Hospital. Getting these two to cooperate would help me win the approval of the Beth Israel Hospital, and so on down the line. I was successful with this "pecking order" strategy, but somewhere down the line a small hospital refused me. It would have made no difference to our final results for they saw so few women with this illness, but I like completeness and decided to try them again. Dr. MacMahon demurred: would people really believe that we got 100 percent cooperation? My compulsion overcame his skepticism; the hospital agreed; we had them all.

It was not smooth sailing even then. Doctors, especially surgeons, are extreme individualists, and I needed endless meetings in each hospital to gain their permission to interview their patients. It was lucky for me that I knew Dr. Oliver Cope. I'd gone to him as a patient soon after our arrival in Boston, and I was tremendously impressed with his wisdom and his humanity. He was the greatly respected chairman of the Department of Surgery at Harvard and chief of surgery at the Mass. General, and he helped to smooth my way.

Just as the pecking order of hospitals intrigued me, so did the pecking order within hospitals. After getting the consent of the director of each hospital and the chief of surgery, I'd ask who I should speak to next, and I'd carry on this way until no more names were mentioned. It was soon clear that hospital medicine, in particular surgery, was dominated by men. No one, in any hospital, suggested that I speak to the director of nursing and her staff! In South Africa as in Britain, matron (chief nurse) was a formidable figure to be ignored at one's peril, and the ward sister always accompanied a doctor on his rounds. Since nurse cooperation was essential for interviewing patients, the more so in rooms housing several patients, I met with them anyway.

It was a mixed blessing to occupy office space on the same floor as Dr. MacMahon. We got extra attention, but also extra assignments—the only center of the seven required to interview home controls. (Essentially, these control cases were women in the Boston area of similar ages to the patients with breast cancer, but without their disease.) While we had no trouble interviewing controls in hospitals, three for each patient, we had real difficulty interviewing women in their homes. Because breast cancer occurs mainly in older women, our controls were also older women. Unfortunately, the "Boston strangler" was on the loose at that time. Anyone who has tried to gain entry into the homes of fearful, elderly women, some of whom have locked themselves into apartments located in seedy areas of the city, will appreciate our problems. We tried every stratagem to get a hearing, but it's hard to be coherent shouting through a grille in an entryway. Twenty percent of the home controls refused to speak to us compared to only 5 percent of the hospital controls. My staff wilted with each refusal.

Staff morale dropped even lower after all the interviewing was finally over. Each center then tried to get figures on the incidence of breast cancer in their area. (The incidence of a disease is the number of *new* cases of that disease within a specified period of time. When the population of the area from which these cases have come is known, a rate can be calculated and compared with that of other areas.) To get the *true* incidence of breast cancer, we needed to find out how many cases we'd missed and add that number to those women we had already counted.

I had chosen a key person in each hospital for us to call at regular intervals to learn when a new case of breast cancer was admitted. The system worked very well, but no system of notification is perfect. When interviewing stopped, we searched the records of the twenty-seven hospitals for the two years we'd worked there to find any missed cases. Before this search began we'd congratulated ourselves on interviewing over 90 percent of all notified cases with this illness. Ironically, the more diligently we searched the records, the more cases we found that had not been notified. With each such discovery the interviewers' excellent record of success diminished and spirits sagged. I emphasized that integrity was the essence of a good study and honesty more important than a high "response rate," but my remarks were poor comfort to staff who were whittling away at their own good efforts. Thankfully, in the final tally, we just reached our goal of interviewing 80 percent of *all* women in our area who were diagnosed as having breast cancer during the two years of our study.[5]

Epidemiologists work hard to disprove their intuitive theories, and they hide their emotions from public view. The reports we wrote for medical journals showed nothing of our underlying tensions, nor conformed in any way to Zinsser's prescription for good writing: humanity, clarity, simplicity, vitality.[6] But I was happy with the work we'd done except for one lasting disappointment. Dr. MacMahon was right, and I was wrong in our predictions. Prolonged breast-feeding had no protective effect against the development of breast cancer. Still, as the Yiddish proverb has it: "Bygone troubles are good to tell."

Transition

The day I got my numbered parking place at the Harvard School of Public Health, I felt settled there. After years of temporary assignments, having an allotted place gave me a sense of stability and belonging. I had a job (I thought) for as long as I wanted to stay and could satisfy myself and my chairman with the work I produced.

In South Africa, at least in my time, nobody spoke of tenure; I had never heard the term. But the day came when my chairman at Harvard told me he'd recommended me for tenure. And the day also came when, to my surprise and chagrin, he had to tell me that the dean of the school had judged me unworthy. I learned that after my eight years in the Department of Epidemiology (three as a research associate, five as a senior research associate), I must either get promoted to a professorial, tenured position or leave Harvard. The dean tempered his ruling by offering me an additional three years in the department if I was willing to start over again as a research associate!

Being rejected bruised my pride and brought back those feelings of inadequacy I had when I first considered working in Boston. I hadn't known how rare female professors were in the Harvard medical establishment[1] or that the first women medical students had been admitted only in 1946. If I'd been a man, I wondered, would the dean have accepted me? I never asked him. To me, he seemed cold and distant, and my contact with him had been limited to once a year at the annual school party where we shook hands in the receiving line and murmured polite "Good evenings."

I took some comfort in the fact that my chairman, who knew me well, had recommended me. And, paradoxically, though I was upset at being forced to leave, I was also somewhat relieved that the decision had been made for me. I was fully convinced of the importance of epidemiologic research, but I'd begun to feel that tackling one research project after another, limited to data measurable in statistical terms and without responsibility for applying my findings, while intellectually satisfying, was emotionally confining. My only reason for staying one more year—as consultant, not research associate—was to finish current work.

The prospect of leaving work unfinished always disturbs me. Twice during my years in epidemiology another university had offered me a job at more than twice my meager Harvard salary, and both times I refused because the timing was wrong. Each time I had been enmeshed in a particular piece of work and felt I *had* to get it done. My chairman airily waved these offers aside by remarking, "It's the work that counts, not the salary." What he really meant was that in his opinion no university could measure up to Harvard. I remember meeting him a year or so after I left his department when he told me I'd made the president's report. I was mystified until it dawned on me that he meant the president of Harvard—the health center I was running at the time had gotten a line or two in that year's Harvard annual report.

Around the time of my rejection at Harvard someone told me that Radcliffe College had started an Institute for Independent Study (now the Bunting Institute). Its purpose was to give older women the chance to change professional fields or get back into academic life after years spent in bringing up children. That Institute could give me exactly what I needed: an opportunity to mull over the direction I should take next. So I met with Constance Smith, the distinguished and kindly head of the program, made my application, and had the good fortune to be accepted as a half-time scholar for a two-year period beginning in the academic year 1966–67. It was understood that I would keep my Harvard appointment during that time in order to complete my epidemiologic research. My acceptance at Radcliffe coincided with the entrance of our daughter, Rosalie, as a freshman; we were Cliffies together—she at sixteen and I at fifty.

Twenty-four women became Radcliffe Scholars that year, joining seventeen others whose appointments had been renewed for a second year. Our fields ranged from arts to anthropology, botany to biology, musicology to medicine, photography to politics. It was a delight to be with so many talented women; I had so often longed for female companionship in academic medicine's predominantly male society—that world that had just wounded me at Harvard.

In my application I asked for time "to acquire a theoretical knowledge and understanding of behavioral patterns of people living in different social settings," because "I wanted to apply that knowledge to community health services—perhaps to community mental health." I wrote, also, that "I needed training in the social and behavioral aspects of medicine, basic sociology, cultural anthropology, community structure and organization." Most importantly, "I needed time to think about the role of health care in communities, the direction I wanted to take, and how to meld the two."

Acceptance at Radcliffe restored a measure of my self-esteem. If I was judged an equal of these able women, I no longer cared as much that the dean had found me lacking. It was our acceptance of each other, the supportive relationships that I now encountered, the lack of pressure and competitiveness, that made the Institute so important to me. Most of us had experienced more difficulty than men do in professional advancement, had seen our careers interrupted more often, had gotten lower pay and less recognition. I was at ease during those weekly seminars as I enjoyed the group warmth and sympathetic interaction. No one showed off her cleverness by scoring points off another, and there was a wonderful feeling of freedom, independence, and trust.

In my mind I compared the women's camaraderie with the competitive attitude of Harvard doctoral students in epidemiology. When these predominantly male students introduced their research projects to staff and peers, their colleagues did not praise the strength of a research design, commend innovation, give encouragement. Instead, seminars became forums at which those who listened could hardly wait to display their erudition by ferreting out each others' weaknesses.

Since I was a student with no specific piece of work to complete for Radcliffe, no special duties to perform, I enjoyed a rare breathing space. I attended some lectures, but mostly I read: cultural anthropology, sociology, social psychology, community mental health. And I joined a creative writing class at Harvard—I had a vague idea even then of writing about my South African experiences in other than scientific journal form. Also I wanted to mix with young people and be stimulated by their fresh ideas. I'd become a little bored with a steady diet of doctors and doctors' wives.

My writing classmates seemed *very* young, but it was fun to listen and enjoy their spontaneity and self-confidence. The teacher, a tall thin dark-haired man, whom I judged to be about five to ten years older than my amiable companions, was also pleasant though a shade nervous. The poor man was in a difficult position since I was old enough to be his mother, and he had problems being too hard on a mother figure.

Whenever he wrote any negative remarks on the manuscripts I handed to him, he made sure to temper his criticism with kindly encouragement. Most often he began with praise and then censured the effort. I would be cheered by a sentence beginning, "This could be developed into a delightful essay or better yet a short-short story." Then came the censure. "What is presently lacking, primarily, is *tone*—the writer is absent, the presentation colorless." He would end by suggesting what I should do about it: choose more "personal" subjects in which I must be totally involved in order to discover style—then tone would follow naturally. But lest I be too discouraged he'd praise the cheerfulness and equanimity of my writing. I felt as sorry for him as I did for myself. When the term ended, he wrote me a sweet letter telling me how he'd been nervous about having me in the class while he expounded to his near contemporaries about the "meaning of life." Again the comforting touch followed, that in fact I'd been a great help in a very difficult seminar. And then came his last advice: suggesting that I make some of my selections almost purely about myself, "or at least strongly imply a world view that is particular and special." I read between the lines. It seemed obvious that what I wrote was so held-in, sketchy, and unrevealing, that I might never be able to write the book I wanted.

Still looking for counsel, I also spent an hour with a pleasant and gentle editor of a prestigious publishing house. He suggested that I write an academic book on "The History of Public Health in America," or, "Medical Care in the Inner City"—the last thing I wanted to do. There was no money in writing, he warned, and joining a class wouldn't teach me how to write. And if I wrote too thinly about myself because I wanted to tell about others, it wouldn't work: readers would want to know about me, not about them. He advised me to write about myself.

I didn't join another creative writing class, but the nagging longing to write on a deeper level surfaced now and again and was hard to suppress completely. Some time before I made up my mind to tackle the present book, I spoke to my son Mark about wanting to write a more personal script, but emphasized how difficult it would be for me to record my own life history. He was sure I could do it. "You've worked with three communities, Mom," he said. "When you write about those people you'll find that you'll also be writing about yourself."

My teacher, the editor and Mark were all right. Even so it took the passage of many years, and my fascination in learning about the lives of others through interviews, before I finally had the courage to write as openly about myself as about the people with whom I worked. While putting this chapter on paper I re-read my early, stiff class efforts, tore them up, laughed at myself, and genuinely appreciated my teacher's kindness.

I was looking forward to a second year at Radcliffe when a Harvard professor I knew socially came to see me. He wanted to interest me in applying for the post of director of a health center in one of Boston's poverty areas. This center was to be placed in a low-income, inner-city housing project on the site of a well-baby clinic run for many years by the Maternal and Child Health Department of the School of Public Health. Support was assured through two grants from the U.S. Government's Children's Bureau. (In the morass of federal funding programs it's enlightening to discover how an individual legislator's family history may determine the purpose of a grant. The Kennedy family became concerned with the field of mental retardation when one of their own was afflicted by this condition. Mental retardation happens more often in premature than in full-term infants; and mothers who are poor, belong to minority groups, and have inadequate prenatal care are more likely to have pre-mature babies.) The purpose of one of the two Children's Bureau grants—the Maternity and Infant Care grant—was to reduce prematurity, and therefore mental retardation, as well as infant mortality, by offering skilled services to pregnant women in poverty populations. The intent of the other—a Children and Youth grant—was to improve the health of deprived children who lived in poverty, again by providing expert attention. Two of Harvard's prestigious teaching hospitals would be responsible for the conduct of the health center. The director of this center would be expected to combine the two programs into a single comprehensive family service for mothers and children and an-swer to a committee of prominent physicians. Many additional administrative details followed before the crucial question came.

Did I want to apply for the position of director of this center?

I felt threatened by this sudden mass of information (after nine years in semisheltered, academic research) and bewildered by the cumbersome administrative system, top heavy as it was with layers of important persons. Questions raced through my mind: How much would these "high-ups" understand about the problems of the poor? How could one organize a family health center when the mandate was to serve only pregnant women and children? Who would care for the women who were not pregnant and for men over the age of twenty-one? Could a third hospital (giving adult services) be approached to fill the gap? If so, what would that do to this already messy administrative tangle? Why were there no community people on a committee overseeing a family health service for poor people? With no theoretical training in health planning and administration, could I learn the necessary skills on the job as I had had to do in epidemiology? Finally, wouldn't I be crazy to give up my second peaceful year at Radcliffe?

If the offer had been to direct a neighborhood health center, I think I would have agreed immediately. My South African experience had convinced me that neighborhood health centers were the cornerstone of community medical care, and I wanted very much to work in a health center setting again. The first U.S. neighborhood health center, at Columbia Point in Boston, had just been established by Jack Geiger, who as a final-year medical student had spent six months in the South African health centers where Harry and I had worked. Dr. Geiger freely acknowledged his use of the South African health center model in fashioning his own centers. But the center I might head was only partially a neighborhood health center and did not speak to the vital issue of community involvement.

Harry had been in the health administration field from his first U.S. job and was at that time the director of a large state hospital. "Where can I get a quick course in health administration?" I asked him. He answered with a laugh that a theoretical course was unlikely to help me. Administration was an art rather than a science, and I got along well with people. I could be an administrator without taking a special course, he said.

I had serious doubts about my ability to meet this new challenge, but my eagerness to become involved with a community on a grass-roots level once again overrode my fears. The decade of the sixties was a time of fervent involvement in the war against poverty, and I'd been sitting on the sidelines in academia. If I missed this opportunity to become engaged, would there be another? I visited the clinic in the housing project and recognized the neighborhood hall where I'd supervised Harvard medical students at some well-baby sessions several years earlier. Somehow that early connection with the place was a cheering omen. If the board wanted me, I would take the job.

One of the requests I made at the time of selection was for a small research unit which I would head. My years in South Africa and in epidemiology had convinced me that I needed to know the fundamental makeup of the "target" population: their numbers, sex, age, race, education, income, employment, and attitudes to health care. Only when I had such information would I be able to plan suitable programs and later measure how well or badly the center reached and served its most needy people. The committee agreed and helped me get separate funding for the research unit—the only unit over which I exercised complete control.

I needed a few months to finish off assignments before I began the job officially as a paid director, but I was too anxious about my lack of knowledge to stay away until I could start full-time employment. Almost immediately I began to read books and seek out advisers who would teach me about Boston's health politics, organization of services, grant programs, housing projects, and the people who lived in them. I met regularly with the core staff of the original well-baby clinic who would continue to work at the center.

It was just as well that my ignorance was a shield. If I had known at the start about the extent of Boston's power politics, its intense racial and religious prejudices, its bureaucratic procedures, its multiple organizations and agencies who fought each other for bigger pieces of the money pie,[2] I might have been scared off and have missed a powerful experience. My two-and-a-half years as director of the center were to be the most turbulent, but in many respects the most rewarding, years of my life.

The Bracken Field Health Center

As director of the Bracken Field Health Center [1]—located in a housing project, and hereafter referred to as the Center—I served a low-income population of pregnant women and children up to age twenty-one who lived in a section of West Hill. When I started my job, I was an unschooled newcomer to the inner-city ghetto and certainly not aware of the divisive bitterness between the people—mostly Irish—who lived outside the housing project and the blacks who lived in it.

Newton, where I lived, was an all-white suburb. To me, American racism, as I saw it on television, was a Southern phenomenon. By and large, South Africans of my generation, black and white, had an idealized conception of American democracy and of black/white relationships. I didn't know about the blatant racism of Northern cities nor of the terrible poverty of "The Other America." [2]

I inherited a well-baby clinic, which had been chosen as a demonstration unit where academic and practical public health knowledge was pooled by staff from Harvard's School of Public Health and public health nurses from the city of Boston. The weekly clinics, however, did little to solve the multiple problems of the housing project population. In the mid-sixties some money from the federal government's antipoverty program allowed the clinic to expand its preventive services [3] and six project apartments were made available to the clinic, but comprehensive services only began six months after I became director of the Center in April 1967. Harvard's Boston Hospital for Women and its Children's Hospital, with support from the U.S. government's Children's Bureau, controlled operations, and I was accountable to a distinguished, male policy committee of representatives from these two hospitals, Harvard Medical School, Harvard School of Public Health, and the Massachusetts State Health Department through which the government grants were funneled.

I saw my role as that of a planner/educator/evaluator. My goal was ambitious—to turn this former well-baby clinic into a neighborhood health center, not just for mothers and children but for all the people of our portion of West Hill. Because I aimed for a neighborhood health center, and because I wanted to improve people's emotional as well as their physical health, I was determined to get the residents of our area actively involved in the policies and planning of the health center.

First I needed to know how many people lived in our target area and what kind of people they were. Fortunately, I had my small research unit, and my first undertaking was the conduct of a door-to-door census of the population.

I'd been looking for temporary summer help for this purpose: young people with energy and spirit, not yet immersed in professional jargon. By chance I found the first one in the waiting room of the Angell Memorial Animal Hospital. Our dog had been run over and had spent some weeks in this hospital. I was taking him for a postoperative check one Saturday morning and was prepared for a long, dull waiting period, when I noticed a young student whose pile of notebooks was crowned by a shoe box with holes in its lid. Conversation with her was an irresistible alternative to bored silence, and I asked about the content of the box. It held her bird, whose leg was broken.

Kay was a first-year law student drawn into that field because of an interest in Spanish rent strikes in Harlem. By the time one of us was called to see the vet, I'd offered her a summer job working on the census. We got together a few more students to help her, in particular, Elsie, a young, talented black girl who vacillated between a future in the white university world and the solidarity of a black separatist group. Our daughter, Rosalie, who volunteered her services, kept the records.

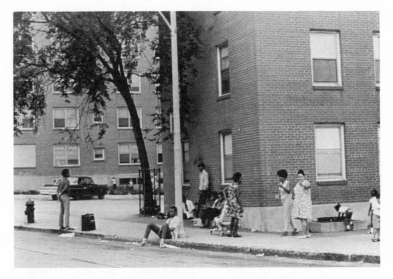

The Bracken Field housing project

We translated information about Medicaid into simple English and Spanish, wrote other brochures about the services we were going to offer, visited local churches, enlisted ministerial support, and gave information to local newspapers. From our analysis of the census survey we calculated that we had a population of 2,000 women of childbearing age and 6,000 children eligible for our services, but ultimately we'd have a population of 17,000 persons when the time came for us to serve everyone— not just pregnant women and children. We learned that ours was a shifting, mobile population—a factor that would add considerably to our patient load.

Our service area lay in West Hill—the housing project being only a part of one section. West Hill is itself a part of Boston and has some beautiful, wooded parkland districts and expensive houses, but in the neighborhood with which we were concerned one fourth of the houses (outside the housing project) were deteriorating or dilapidated. The rest were modest homes of poor or lower-middle-income families. Two-thirds of these homes were rental housing. West Hill was almost entirely white, Irish, Catholic with a small though rapidly increasing Hispanic stream and a few Greek and Italian families.

This white area encased a predominantly black pocket—a low-income housing project which I call Bracken Field. I chose this name partly in irony because city fathers so often name slummy streets "sunrise" or "sunset" or other equally ludicrous title. My description of the scene is the way I saw it in April 1967.

Bracken Field was one of the largest housing projects in Boston. A mix of seven-story and three-story blocks, it was as ugly and devoid of grace as all these high-rise projects seemed to be. The few trees were protected from humans by iron palings. Red brick buildings, all alike, surrounded courtyards of concrete and asphalt. The young were provided with a tot-lot containing the usual swings and slides, but its base of concrete was littered with broken bottles and rusted cans. Incinerators were provided but were too small; children sent to empty the garbage dumped the excess in hallways and gutters. Broken windows were a common sight, but worse than these were boarded windows because they signified a fire, injury, perhaps death. Stairs and hallways were dark, for light bulbs were often stolen or broken, yet elevators were avoided in the seven-story blocks for fear of mugging.

I *hated* the project for its ugliness, its cheerlessness, its barracklike quality, its anonymity. There was little pride of ownership in these apartments, since tenants preferred to feel that their stay in them was temporary. Apartments were numbered, but bore no names, knockers, or peepholes. Mailboxes in the vestibules were regularly smashed on the first and fifteenth days of each month when the welfare checks arrived; eventually our collective complaints resulted in checks being dispatched on a less predictable schedule. There was a neighborhood hall but no laundromat, no shop, no supermarket in the project itself.

People who lived here did so from necessity, not choice. In the old days they got into public housing by applying to their

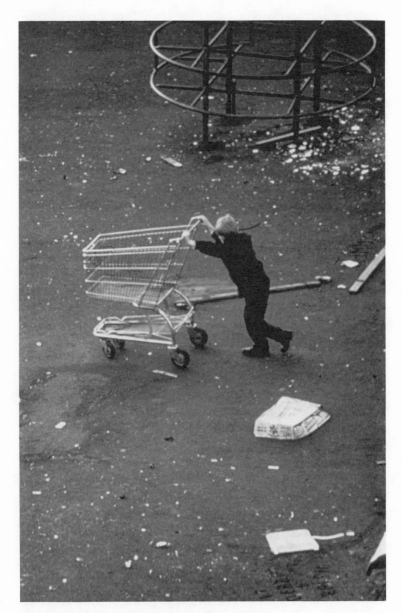

Playtime could be hazardous

legislative representatives; later they got in through the dispensation of the social services department. Since only the poor qualified for subsidized housing, all who entered were poor. But there were always more poor people than rental housing units, so poverty alone was insufficient. Most who came had multiple problems. The vast majority were black, and in most families fathers were either absent, sick, or disabled. There were many young children; 40 percent of all children in our area lived there. Sixty percent of project families subsisted on welfare payments. It was a world of troubled mothers with children to support.

One of the housing authority's rules was that once families earned over a certain amount of money they must leave their subsidized apartments. This rule undoubtedly was made with good intent to free low-rental apartments for the most needy. At the same time it meant that people who were successful, who achieved, who were looked up to by others, who were the "Joneses" (as Mark Clay put it to me later), were told to leave. As a result children grew up in a dreary atmosphere of failure. Amazingly, a handful of remarkable families who earned more than the maximum somehow managed to stay. They were admired and respected as leaders in the community.

Few families in Bracken Field made deep friendships on either side of the color line. Suspicion, mistrust, fear of thieves, drug addicts, and muggers was rife. The families lived side by side with equally bereft strangers. One section of Bracken Field was set aside for the elderly poor—most of them white. They lived an indoor life, afraid to venture out for fear of mugging. To place defenseless old people in such high-crime areas as a solution to their poverty made one despair of the sensitivity of those who make our laws and regulations. It defied understanding.

I discussed the nature of housing projects with an extraordinary staff member: Sister Patricia, our psychiatric social worker and a nun of the order of St. Vincent de Paul. She and her nun companion (a teacher) had tremendous courage. They chose to live in the project, discarding the protection of their nuns' garb.

After they were mugged, they wore the headdress of their order, but only after working hours. "When we were mugged we immediately called the police, but they didn't come. We called again and explained to the Irish cop that we were Roman Catholic nuns, thinking this would certainly make them come, but it didn't. And when we first moved in I went to cash a check in the supermarket. I showed my driver's license and asked for a courtesy card. The man in the booth had no idea who I was. He said, "Oh Pattie, babe, we don't give courtesy cards here. This is only welfare and factory people."

Sister Patricia told me that before moving into Bracken Field she'd thought of poverty as a lack of food and clothing, but now it meant living in a poor neighborhood as helpless victims of crime and violence. Nobody really cared about the poor in America, she said, because if they did the lives of the poor would be very different. The major problems of the area were not health problems in the simple sense. The residents wanted our center to agitate for police protection, better housing, better maintenance, rat extermination, and recreational facilities. They wanted centers for child day-care, for mentally retarded children, for treatment of drug addicts. As director of the health center I felt all these concerns were legitimate community health issues and part of my job to address.

Within a year of starting full services more than half of all eligible families had registered with us as patients—even though those who lived outside the project were afraid when they had to come there to see us. In the project itself most of the eligible families had registered. We overflowed the six apartments allotted to us in our three-story block. Staff clamored for the remaining six apartments of the block we were in, but I demurred at the thought of evicting tenants. Meeting with these tenants I explained our predicament. What did they think I should do? Their answers surprised me and strengthened my belief in asking before acting. They all wanted to leave those particular apartments: sharing a block with a clinic meant constant traffic, noise, vandalism. They'd move gladly if and when we got them other apartments—especially if they had an extra bedroom.

We weren't allowed to make any architectural changes that couldn't be reversed if we moved out. Usually public buildings have too few bathrooms (except in South Africa where the government provides toilets for whites, browns, and blacks), but in the Center we had too many bathrooms as well as too many kitchens and were hard put to make the best use of them. In the summer the buildings were very hot. I toyed briefly with the idea of putting an air conditioner in my bedroom office, but resisted the temptation because I didn't want to be treated differently from everyone else, and because it was sure to be stolen. At one time we installed an inexpensive burglar alarm; the wires were cut within a week—our center was fair game. Eventually we hired two residents as security guards, one for daytime, the other for nighttime hours, but even this did not fully solve our problems.

As far as I can recall, I made only three inviolable rules for the clinical practice: staff would work as members of teams, nobody could smoke in front of a patient, and no student could examine a patient without prior permission from his preceptor *and* the patient. This was a time when communities, especially black communities, were complaining bitterly that they were being used as guinea pigs for students. I remember asking consent at a community meeting for medical students to rotate through our clinics, explaining that each student would have to get prior permission. I made the point that if the community wanted to have doctors who were sympathetic to the plight of the poor, students would have to be exposed to poverty populations. My request was put to a vote and agreed upon.

One particularly pleasant medical student, Craig, asked to spend a summer field placement at our Center. Since I was too busy to carve out chunks of time for him, I suggested that he share my office and be with me at all my appointments. In the ten days he spent with me, I asked each person I met whether Craig could be present. (At the merest sign of hesitation, he would disappear.) In this way he heard about neighborhood protests against building an expressway through our area, the latest mugging, the constant presence of roaches, the dumping of an abandoned car in our parking area, the drop-out rate at school, the futile search for decent jobs, the poor lighting and lack of police protection, as well as more mundane clinical problems. After a few days I took Craig to sit in at a regular team meeting during which selected families were discussed. At one point in the discussion I leaned over and whispered to him, "They didn't teach us this kind of thing in medical school." Craig looked at me in amazement. "Are you a *doctor?*" he asked in a tone of utter disbelief. It was an important insight into medical school training for both of us.

For all that, when Dan, a politically aware, second-year Harvard medical student, came to the Center to ask my opinion about his intention to quit school and become a community organizer, I advised against it. I thought he'd be more useful to the people he wanted to help if he finished his studies. (The fact that students ask for counsel doesn't at all mean they will take the advice they came for. Often, they simply voice their ambivalences aloud to people who'll listen sympathetically.) Dan did drop out for two years while he worked with a community not far from our own but then returned to school and became a family practitioner. Now he directs a rural health clinic in a depressed coal-mining town and is happy in his work. From time to time he calls me, ostensibly to get my opinion or to ask for a reference, but mostly to report progress and to keep in touch. His enthusiasm is a tonic on days when I feel my age.

Sometimes the boost from the past is completely unexpected. When we moved to North Carolina and I was working at Duke, the university was trying very hard to entice a well-known academic physician to head a new department. Harry and I were invited to one of the parties Duke gave in honor of this prospective candidate. I didn't know the candidate but was introduced to him by the chairman of my department. The guest smiled and told me that, though I didn't know him, he knew me. He had been one of the students passing through my Center, and it had left an indelible impression. Such incidents, rare as they are, are sweet rewards.

We divided our geographic area between two teams: one to be responsible for the people of Bracken Field, the other for the people outside the project. Doctor, nurse, and social worker were the essential team members. The psychiatrist, group worker, nutritionist, and dentist served both teams. I wanted to add community aides to the teams. Aides were residents of our target area and at first were only used by the nurses as baby-sitters so mothers could keep appointments. I felt they were wasted as sitters for they knew and could teach us the *real* problems of the families we discussed. And coming to team meetings would educate the aides in matters of health, making them more effective in their community.

I believed strongly that employing residents in as many positions as possible, with on-the-job training, was one important way to get community involvement, raise community self-esteem, and give residents needed income. It also made the clinic a friendlier place for patients, helped us learn community proprieties, and integrated professional and lay staff. It took a while before these neighborhood aides were accepted at team meetings, but they proved their worth.

One aide discussed with me the troublesome question of the right to enter a tenant's apartment uninvited. Who, if anybody, had such a right? Our public health nurses had visited homes long before the initiation of our health center. They never questioned their own entries but resented other personnel visiting *their* families. I sympathized with the aide's feelings when she complained to me. "Well, I always thought that aides had been used somewhat as peeping toms for nurses and for Social Service—they almost expect them to be some kind of an information bureau for their use. I say, don't force yourself on anybody. I think people should be *invited* into homes." On the other hand, she conceded that she wanted me and others to know and understand the problems that existed, and home visits were necessary to get such knowledge. I did visit homes, always getting prior permission, sometimes accompanying a nurse or an aide, other times alone. In these apartments there were no books, the few pictures I saw were crude religious depictions, and television supplied constant background noise.

Another aide, who had grown up in rural North Carolina, described to me how painful it had been for her when public welfare social workers would not sit in her chair—showing her they felt it would be dirty. "In the ghetto we always saw social workers as people coming to ask us for papers. You sign this and you tell me that and where is your insurance papers?" I remember her expression when she told me, "Most people don't know what it is to be poor. It's hard to tell the feel of hunger." Life in a ghetto meant having people "looking at us like we was worms, and they was studying us." She confided to me that at first people had asked her how I could care about them since I was white. It had taken her time to learn that I really did care, and we talked intimately about North Carolina and her own family's prejudice against Jews, which she had accepted without thought.

At times professional and lay staff could not work together. The white, medical record librarian was a stickler for accuracy, neatness, and punctuality—all essential ingredients for this job—but the black, assistant medical records clerk, an intelligent, friendly talkative soul, lacked these particular attributes. The librarian issued an ultimatum: one or the other had to go. Since both were valuable people, and I wasn't prepared to lose either of them, I carefully reassigned the clerk to another clerical position with an increase in pay. However the Health Advisory Committee (commonly known as HAC and about whom I will have much to say later) decided that I should have dismissed the librarian and came to me to complain. I met with the committee, and the matter seemed to be resolved amicably. But nothing is simple in a deprived, suspicious community. The chairman of HAC—at that time white—reported to me that certain black members voiced the sentiment that I must, after all, be a racist. I told the chairman that if by this time they didn't know I was *not* a racist, nothing I could say would convince them, and she shouldn't spend time worrying over it.

We had problems also about the qualifications of residents for advertised jobs. The local antipoverty, Area Planning Action Committee (APAC), wanted to place as many residents as possible in jobs with us, and we worked closely together. To APAC placing someone who'd recently been released from jail was a triumph. But to us such reasons were not sufficient; for example, a secretary must also be able to type.

The complexity of our organizational setup was clearly demonstrated in our nursing pool with its clinic nurses, specialist nurses and public health nurses, and the large network of social service agencies in Boston was even more complicated than the nursing scene. Just as families had had more than one nurse visiting their homes, so there could easily be two or even three social service agencies working on different problems and with different family members. We were lucky that the caliber of our nurses and social workers was so high that they overcame those administrative tangles, but at times I was amazed that we functioned as well as we did.

Our clinical staff all had appointments at one or other of our two Harvard hospitals. One clinical appointment that I made was unusual for these centers at this time. It made no sense to me to separate physical and mental health, the more so in situations where so many patients suffered from both ills, so it was a good day when we appointed a part-time community psychiatrist whom I'd known at Harvard. There was no way Ian could diagnose or treat all our clients—the load was overwhelming. Rather, his role was to educate our primary staff so they could handle their patients' emotional problems in addition to their physical.

Our administrative, secretarial, and research staff were an engaging group. But the first administrator chosen by our parent hospitals was a rather stiff Asian, very conscious of his authority and quite unused to our relaxed behavior and to the culture of poverty. I was surprised to find that he kept his briefcase locked, though when he unlocked it in my presence all I could see in it was a copy of *Time* magazine. He was obsequious to me and lordly to underlings; in the words of his staff, "He licked up and kicked down." The poor man was obviously misplaced and didn't last long, but his successor was genial, competent, and ambitious; he outlasted me. Several of the group could have fitted well into the Peace Corps; they'd chosen to work with a poverty population, and they were demanding of me and of themselves.

The administrative secretary had a master's degree in English and wrote poetry. A longtime activist, she sent me regular notes complaining of our slow pace and urging more determined measures toward community involvement, but she also sent several supportive messages such as: "E.J.S. I've just decided that you cannot leave Bracken Field." My personal secretary, Amy, who grew to know me better than anyone outside of my immediate family, was a gentle idealist. Her friend, Brenda, secretary to the nursing division, became my successor's secretary when Amy insisted on following me to my next job. I give an account of Brenda, told to me by an aide, to convey the spirit of this unusual group.

"Brenda come down one day and say she going to jail. I say, what you going to jail for? She say, the people come out of the health center and can step right into this big hole in the street here and the city they don't fix it. She say, I done call to city hall, and I tell them I got a wrench ready, and if they don't have someone here by 10:15 today, I'm going to break the fire hydrant! I say, you sure is going to jail. Then I tell her, it's my community, you don't live here, I'll go to jail, not you. She say, no, she going to jail 'cos people here is human beings, and if the hole was in Stoughton, Brookline, or Wellesley, they'd have fixed it long ago. So I tell the other aides, and they all say if Brenda go to jail we all go. So sure enough we all sitting there waiting for the time to come to break the hydrant. About three minutes before 10:15 Public Works come out and fill that hole up. So we don't go to jail."

Our clinic manager was Kay, whom I'd hired to organize the original household census survey. At the end of that summer

Kay announced that she wasn't going back to law school; she wanted to stay with me. She promised to do anything I asked of her: type, scrub floors, anything at all. She became the clinic manager, and later, when we needed to replace our community organizer, she took that on and did just as well.

I knew nothing of Kay's family background at the time I hired her and didn't inquire, but that year the American Public Health Association met in her hometown, and her parents invited Harry and me to dinner. Her father, I discovered, owned a chain of newspapers, a television station, and a football team. When Kay and I were back at the center, I asked her why her parents had honored me in this fashion when I was employing their daughter in a ghetto, and I wanted to know why Kay had come to work for me. "Some people are born with a silver spoon in their mouth," she said; "I was born with a gold spoon."

Though Kay was worth her weight in gold to me, some of the older staff objected to the responsibility I gave to one so young and lacking in experience. Besides, she wore miniskirts. I listened to their objections, smoothed ruffled feathers, but kept Kay with me. Some years later, she visited me in Chapel Hill, before I'd started working. When I asked her to go with Philip to pick daffodils for the house, she looked at me strangely. "This is the woman I worked with in the housing project," she complained to Philip. "Daffodils indeed! What your mother needs is a job."

Our research workers were equally hardworking. Two of the four part-time interviewers of my Harvard breast-cancer team joined us at the Center—one was far left politically, the other the wife of a minister, who at the time was in Mississippi fighting for integration. I've already mentioned Elsie who'd started with the census and later became my research assistant. (In the end I lost Elsie to her black separatist group.) Our statistician, kindly and reliable, got on well with everyone. All were part-time (my research grant was small), underpaid, and exceptional people.

I've talked at some length about our staff because they were such fine people and because a neighborhood health center can't succeed without idealism, competency, and teamwork.

The policy committee left me very much to my own devices. We were supposed to meet monthly, but often some members would be absent. The first few meetings took place in a hospital boardroom, an incongruous atmosphere of calm and plenty far removed from the violence and poverty of the people whose health we were discussing. (Boardrooms with their power and opulence do make me feel uncomfortable, but until recently I had a sneaking liking for their huge, beautiful wood tables. When I saw a photograph of a black cleaning woman kneeling on top of a boardroom table in Johannesburg and polishing it by hand, even the tables lost their appeal.)[4] After these first few months the committee agreed that we'd meet at the health center. I wanted them to experience, at least once a month, our grim and grimy environs. Between meetings I sent them memos outlining what I'd done since the last meeting and what I proposed to do before the next one. Since these memos went unanswered, I took their silence for consent and proceeded on my way.

At one meeting I asked that a community representative be appointed to the committee and named Mark Clay as a well-qualified person. My suggestion was accepted with remarkably little discussion, and I was elated for Mark had become my friend and mentor. In his understated manner, he taught me more about community involvement than anyone else before or since. He did so much for me that it gave me great pleasure to steer him away from his dead-end, arduous factory job to, what he called, "a job with dignity" as director of community relations at Children's Hospital. It is a measure of the man that while his supervisor regarded that job as director of *black* community relations, Mark refused to make racial distinctions. His advice to me on how to get community participation was simple and direct: "Be visible." It took me a while to realize that people had to see me as a familiar figure at meetings, at festivities, and generally around the neighborhood. They had to recognize me and learn to trust me if we were to work together.

The first time I saw Mark Clay in action he'd just been elected president of APAC, and he ran the meeting with good humor and

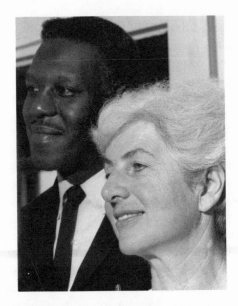

With community leader and mentor Mark Clay

confidence. I was much impressed. Later, I learned that Mark spent as much time in the APAC office, unpaid, as he did in his paid factory job. He told me without embarrassment how he'd read the antipoverty guidelines over and over, sweated over procedure, and studied "Robert's Rules of Order." APAC members met every fortnight, always at night; it was the first of a growing number of organizational meetings which took me away from home after normal working hours.

Once I'd met Mark, I sought his advice freely, and he was always patient with me. His wife, a fine woman, became a community activist in order to see more of him! She told me he was the most patient man in the world—a characteristic I found singularly lacking in many other leaders. Mark was a big man, tall and heavy-set, with a ready smile. His life had been hard (it included a prison term for nonsupport of a child later proven not to be his), but he wasn't bitter or revengeful. He enjoyed his status in the housing project and never wanted to leave it because he was a role model for the youth of Bracken Field.

On the other hand, Ed Gray, another community leader, made life difficult. His thinking appeared convoluted, his manner abrasive, his demeanor depressed. He certainly lacked Mark's open personality. I wasn't aware of Ed's existence, or that of the Modernization Committee which he chaired, until on the third day of June, I got this telegram from him. "Urgent. That the Policy Making Board of the Medical Center meet with the Bracken Field Modernization Committee on June 6th at 1 p.m., at 30 Brick Street, Room 65. Ed Gray." I called his committee office at all hours for the next two days, and Ed's house at night, leaving messages with his wife, but got no response from him. On Mark's advice, I sent a telegram back, learning that this was a common way to communicate in the project! I told Ed Gray that I alone would meet with him and the members of his committee at the appointed time; it was impossible to get my policy committee members together at such short notice.

The meeting with Ed Gray and three of his committee members—in an office across the street from our Center!—lasted three hours. During that time he lambasted me for what "You white people have done to black Americans." I had enough personal guilt feelings about South African whites' behavior to South African blacks not to want to take on another country's guilt, and I denied my involvement. That made matters worse. He asked where I was from and, though I longed to say Newton, Massachusetts, I told the truth and explained our reasons for leaving our country. Ed literally spat out the words "South Africa" and began to attack me personally.

Why was the health center employing white, highly qualified, degree people instead of black residents? Why were we not giving services to adults? Why had we put a service in place without prior consultation with the residents? Why had we decided to name the Center after a white woman? I sympathized with much of what he said but could not persuade him of my limited powers or of the curbs imposed by Children's Bureau guidelines. He talked about a "long hot summer," riots which had taken place in several U.S. cities, rising black anger, and ended with a veiled threat of "Molotov cocktails" in our area. Ed's last words to me were that he'd put me through "sensitivity training" and that he'd do the same with my staff. He hadn't succeeded in reducing me to tears, but my legs trembled as I crossed the road to go back to my office. It was the only time in my life when I felt that a strong dose of whiskey might not be a bad idea.

In subsequent months Ed Gray called me several times to complain of staff shortcomings in patient care. Each time I promised to investigate, found the complaints to be groundless, and reported back politely. Then, on one awful day a child was bitten twice by rats. The project was in an uproar, and the Modernization Committee called for a community meeting that night. I longed not to go back to yet another night meeting, but this was a very serious matter, and there was no way I could stay home. I remember saying to Harry that if I went to the meeting people would be pleased to see me, but would forget my previous attendances if I missed the next meeting. They'd say, "You see, she's not here; she doesn't care." They *were* pleased to see me and laughed when I said they'd better give me an apartment in the project since I spent so much of my time there.

As soon as he saw me, Ed Gray hit out at me. "It's all your fault," he told me angrily. "Why is it my fault?" I asked. "It's your fault because you're not treating people's minds. If you treated people's minds as well as their bodies," he said, "they'd keep their apartments clean, and they wouldn't throw garbage out of the window. The rats wouldn't breed like they do now, and they wouldn't bite the children. It's all your fault." I answered his charges and kept my cool, but no logical reply can overcome the frustrations of a long-neglected community. Fortunately, I had arranged for city sanitarians to be at the meeting and an extermination program (rats and roaches) was arranged which helped for a short while.

When I reported the rat incident and meeting to the policy committee, one member wanted to know why I'd gone to the meeting at all. (By this time, with the encouragement of the state office, our Center was paying the salary of a community advocate as staff for HAC.) He insisted it was her job to go to community meetings, not mine. I disagreed. It was her job, and it was my job too. He was not convinced.

In April 1968 Dr. Martin Luther King, Jr., was assassinated, and our area was in an uproar. Our parent hospitals, afraid for our safety, thought it wise policy to close the clinic, temporarily, until conditions improved. I was uneasy about the wisdom of this decision and asked APAC's opinion. "You can close," they told me, "but if you do, don't think you will ever be able to reopen." The policy committee then agreed we could stay open provided that only staff who volunteered their services be expected to come to work. Community people were convinced we'd come to no harm at work, but there might be problems getting to and from the Center, and patients as well as staff might be stranded there. Children's Hospital arranged transportation for us for a week or so and supplied us with several days of food. Staff drew up emergency plans, stretchers and equipment were supplied, and morale was high. Mark Clay borrowed our Center's van, tied a white display rag to it, and drove around the area cooling angry feelings. It was touch and go, but we remained open and came to no harm.

All the same, anxiety abounded. For many months the project was abuzz with rumors—resembling George Eliot's huge whispering-gallery—and the black population was bitter and hostile to whites. There were mutterings of discontent about the coming dedication ceremony when the Center would be named after a white pediatrician. Questions were surfacing; why were we not naming the Center after Martin Luther King?

A week before our June dedication day, two staff members, one white and one black, came to report phone calls they'd gotten about impending trouble at the dedication. What trouble?

A bomb would go off! And who was behind this? Ed Gray and a youth worker close to him. I was in a quandary. Should I call off the dedication at this very late stage? If I didn't and a bomb exploded, I would be responsible. In the end I decided to confront Ed directly. So I walked to his house, told him the rumor, and asked if there was any truth in it. Ed was completely taken aback and very angry. He declared it was terrible for people to accuse him in this fashion; he was not a man of violence. I believed him (though I remembered his talk of Molotov cocktails), but I needed to know whether there was likely to be any violence at the ceremony. He told me there was always likely to be trouble in a community like ours; a little incident could trigger a riot, but he, certainly, was not going to make trouble. When I pleaded for his help, he suggested I call a meeting of all the men in the project and ask them to lend a hand in keeping things calm at the ceremony. The men agreed and asked that, in turn, I and other female members of my staff sell baseball tickets for them on the great day. (Not much feminist sentiment in this community.) Following Mark's advice, I also arranged for two plainclothes black policemen to be present.

I was extremely worried about the safety of the crowd, including the frail, elderly lady for whom the Center was being named. Half in jest I told some staff members that I was going to buy the brightest dress in Boston; if anyone was to be clearly marked, it had better be me than our distinguished visitor. When I appeared on the special day clad in a bright yellow, floral dress, I heard a voice greeting me: "Here comes the target!"

The day started very badly. The Center had been broken into during the previous night and once again typewriters had been stolen. At that point I was very near to giving up. But the rest of the day was a great success, and everyone was happy. Kay had gotten contributions from local merchants and a $500 donation from her father. She used part of this windfall to hire a marquee (erected in our parking area), to rent tables as booths for the local organizations and agencies who wanted to publicize

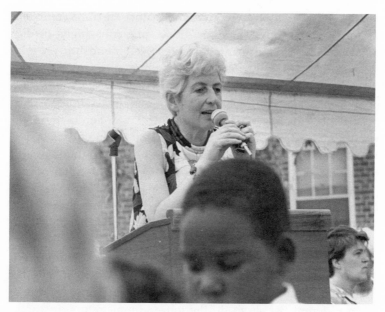

Dedication day: The target

their objectives (HAC had been working on their material for months), and to put up a podium for the speakers.

We ordered 4000 ice creams (hoodsies), cases of Cokes, loads of cakes and cookies, nine urns of coffee—a lift for the morale of a deprived community. And "Mothers for Action," a Bracken Field women's group cooked thousands of hot dogs. Philip, who came with Harry, marveled that we also served watermelon at a predominantly black affair. And we hired a band aptly named "The Consolers."

I introduced Harry and Philip to Ed Gray, and we chatted amiably until Ed spotted a reporter. Immediately, he told me he was going to bring up complaints against the Center. We didn't clear the rubbish in Bracken Field, we let children find and use old syringes in the rubbish, etc. At first I begged that he not spoil our lovely day, but he was adamant, and I got angry. I told him it was not *our* responsibility to remove the rubbish nor the snow in winter (a frequent complaint). He could complain as much as he wanted; I simply didn't care. Amazingly, he did not complain, and we maintained a reserved friendship. He told me once that I was a leader in their community, and I replied that he, too, was a leader; we were partners in both wanting to build up Bracken Field. Of course, being Ed, he wouldn't accept the partnership. I wanted very much to know him better and, later, asked his permission to include him among the people I hoped to interview for my book. At first he refused, then agreed, but didn't keep his appointment. In the end I decided not to pursue him; it was kinder to respect his ambivalence. To misquote Grace Paley: It wasn't his ocean I was a wave in.

For our guest we had prepared a beautiful photograph album of pictures of staff and patients, with my captions and dedication message. Strung together, the captions read: "Communication involves trust, understanding and affection between adults; Communication is looking after little boys and girls; It takes a lot of different people to do the job—administrators, research personnel, social workers, secretaries, aides, nurses, dental staff, doctors—all dedicated to the community, especially to the children; We are settling down to bridge the communication gap by gaining the trust of the residents in the area we serve and working with them in their roles of staff members, parents, and advisers to the health facility; Communication with the poor is fundamentally the same as communication with your next door neighbor; You simply recognize them as human." Our guest was visibly touched. She said she had been in every state of the nation, but never had she been happier with an honor than with this one.

From that party we went to another, given by one of Harry's staff doctors at the Shattuck Hospital. The host had a home with enough parkland to enclose the whole housing project. On his grounds was a beautiful swimming pool; in his basement a model train set with mountains, a ski lift, a waterfall, all operated by computer. How impossible it seemed for the world I worked in to reach the world I visited in.

The repeated thefts of our Center's equipment had become a horrendous problem since we didn't have money for easy re-placement. After the dedication I called a community meeting and told the assembly we'd have to move the Center out of Bracken Field if such thefts continued. Did they suspect, as I did, that the culprits were adolescents hooked on drugs? If that was the case, residents made things worse by buying stolen goods from these children.

The reaction was immediate and impassioned. Bracken Field had a bad drug problem—all the mothers feared for their sons but didn't know what to do about it. That night they began to plan a community-run drug unit, with medical backup from the health center and from the community mental health center into whose area we fell. When the drug unit finally began to operate (after my time), two ex-drug addicts acted as its therapists.

After I left the Center, I interviewed the two therapists—Mario and Cecil. Mario had stayed clean, but during my interview with Cecil he asked me to buy him an ice cream at the drugstore below my new office. A short while after resuming the interview, Cecil began to "nod," though he continued to give me his life history. When he was ready to leave, he conned me into buying a carved walking stick he'd crafted. I was willing to pay my dues for the interview, but when he came back next morning with a crudely carved head, I didn't succumb. I made a second appoint-ment with Cecil for the following week at 3:00 P.M., but he called that afternoon to say he was delayed at a meeting and couldn't see me till 6:00 P.M. Mario had warned me. "As a doctor I would ask you to help people understand what a junkie is. He's a very dangerous person. He'll trick you, he'll steal from you. You have your hand out and you turn your head, he'll take your hand too." I was not about to be alone in a building with Cecil and canceled the appointment. I was no longer a member of the drug committee, or of the health center, but I was worried about Cecil and called my successor to alert him about my suspicions, since our move to North Carolina was imminent. Soon I was immersed in a new place, and for many years I forgot about Cecil.

Ten years later, while visiting Brooklyn and riding the subway, I suddenly remembered Cecil as I sat opposite a black man who was obviously stoned. A tall, sturdily built man, he was wearing soiled clothes, canvas shoes that didn't match, and one old glove tied around his wrist with a rubber band. His eyes were closed, and as the train jerked, he keeled from side to side never quite reaching the seat with his head. Riders on either side of him moved as far away as possible to make sure they didn't become his pillow. Gradually, he recovered consciousness, and he left the train before I did. Passengers mouthed an audible sigh of relief. I thought about Cecil and about how far a doctor's responsibility extends, but I didn't know the answer, then or now.

At this time community residents rarely controlled neighborhood health centers. The common pattern was professional control. I favored a partnership between the two, though I didn't know of any models of this kind. But many road blocks stood in the way.

First, when the parent hospitals decided to expand the clinic into a health center (without discussing their plans with neighborhood people), residents' expectations were far too high. They hoped the Center would be open day and night, that doctors would visit homes, that the whole family would be served, that day-care and other such facilities would appear overnight. They hoped, too, that environmental conditions would improve, maintenance would be better, rats and roaches would disappear, drug addiction and alcoholism would vanish.

Our staff were equally unrealistic. Kenneth Clark has pointed out that social scientists, social workers, and teachers (I would add doctors) are not trained to understand the complex realities of ghetto populations.[5] Mostly young, idealistic, and caring, the staff knew little of the politics of health care. Few were really familiar with the culture of a crisis-oriented population who lived from day to day paying no heed to preventive care or to appointment dates and times. Though they had chosen to work with a poverty group, staff resented militant, aggressive patients who talked back.

Unlike professional staff, community residents employed at the Center were not accustomed to middle-class standards of punctuality. Many had not held steady jobs and were not used to a work routine. Difficulties with child-care arrangements also made for frequent absences.

While the gap between professional and nonprofessional staff was wide, the gap between professionals and community residents was immense. Few ever met socially; contacts were usually limited to dispensing and receiving services. Professionals who could not see patients as citizens found it hard to accept community people as participatory decisionmakers.

On the other hand, community people, whose knowledge of professional expertise was meager, simplified job roles and believed they could replace many professionals (except physicians) with a minimum of training. Reasoned dialogue between the two sides was, at times, replaced by hidden anger on the part of professionals and shouting on the part of residents. Seldom did they truly listen to each other. I believed the professionals should be the more patient, for the cards were stacked in their favor. Most residents in the project had absorbed society's image of them as failures, and many reacted to their problems with apathy, inadequacy, and helplessness. It was a difference of class as much as race.

I tried to bring people closer together through a long-range educational effort aimed at the parent hospitals, Center staff, and community residents. Our entire staff met once a month for lunch-time discussions with outside persons. We had speakers from Boston's mayoral offices (it was the time of "Little City Halls"), from Model Cities, the Martin Luther King neighborhood health center in the Bronx, from Boston's police community relations program, from Boston's prominent black councillor, Tom Atkins, and from faculty of several Boston universities. Our most distinguished overseas guests were Sir George Godber, first Chief Medical Officer of the British National Health Service (who thought it was terrible that we had to fight so hard to get funding for our services), and Dr. Cicely Williams, the famous pediatrician who did so much work with kwashiorkor babies in Africa. I invited HAC members to these meetings, but they never came. They were more comfortable in the program designed specifically for them.

My greatest effort in getting community involvement was to establish a committee of residents to advise the Center. I knew that an ignorant lay committee could never stand up to professionals; committee members would need a long period of careful preparation before they could hope to be accepted as partners. From the day I became director, I recruited possible members to HAC—by word of mouth through census workers, clinic personnel, community organizations, and the distribution of flyers. Response was slow at first, and meetings were held only once a month. But when membership reached twenty (mostly women), and we met twice weekly, I felt cautiously optimistic. But by now I was spending so much of my time with HAC that I decided to use one of the unfilled social work positions to hire a community organizer. Together we designed an elaborate ongoing curriculum of education, part of the training to be done by the antipoverty agency.

At our center we concentrated on health matters. HAC members met with each of our departments to learn their functions. I screened with them every research proposal that we, or others, wanted to try out in our area. We also arranged field trips to our parent and other Boston hospitals, to neighborhood health centers, and other centers like ours. HAC members began receiving invitations to speak to students; some attended conferences. For at least eight women membership in HAC became a central interest in their lives. When Celia Holder became HAC's chairman, she got numerous requests to serve on a variety of consumer committees.

But all this took time to accomplish. It took me fifteen months of pushing before HAC members felt strong enough to agree with me that I must step down as their chairman. I told them they had to fight me to get what they wanted. They couldn't do that if I was chairman; it was a conflict of interests. One of HAC's members, Stella Jones, told my secretary, Amy, that I nurtured HAC as she, herself, nurtured the tomato seeds she grew. I was also chairman of APAC's health committee, but they were more self-assured and pragmatic than HAC—my job was to teach them how to manage without me, and when I'd done that, they'd tell me to step down.

Inevitably, as their confidence grew, HAC members stepped on professionals' toes. When they began criticizing doctors, dentists, and social workers, we were in trouble. Part of the problem was that I hadn't taken staff with me each step of the way and had too freely assumed like thinking. Even loyal supporters were upset with the extent of power they saw me giving to "psychopaths, bad mothers, irresponsible people." I remember replying that I didn't want to see their clinical records; my relationship with them was one of citizen to citizen.

HAC came into its own when I resigned in October 1968. The Center had done very well in its first year of Children's Bureau funding, and I left, happily, on vacation. During my absence someone in the state office or in Children's Bureau (bureaucracy is faceless) decided that we didn't need certain staff positions and subtracted the cost of their salaries, plus money for miscellaneous other items, from the total budget. In the letter from the state office I was informed that I could, within the limits of the figure they allowed (a sum less than our first year's budget), rearrange the budget. It was an unexpected shock, particularly since we found out that the budget of a sister Children and Youth project had not been cut. (In fact within a week of my announcing my resignation, I got a letter from the medical director of that sister project offering me a job; presumably he had money to spare.)

I did rewrite the budget—cutting raises of senior personnel, doing away with the "walk-in" doctor (who saw patients without appointments) not replacing staff who'd left, changing several full-time to half-time positions, delaying essential renovations, and cutting down on weekend hours of service. But it was a bitter blow, which I felt to be unjust and unmerited since we'd done more, not less, than we'd promised. After I'd rearranged the budget in such a way that we could survive as a center for the following year, I resigned. There are times when a job is not as important as a protest. Since, however, the Center and the community were dear to me, I said I'd stay until a new director was appointed—almost a year later. When he came on board, he had no difficulty in getting a substantially increased budget for the following year.

My resignation transformed HAC. They sent a letter to Children's Bureau stating their displeasure at the Center's budget cut and citing the lack of prior consultation on the budget action. They also went to a hearing in Washington, met with representatives of Children's Bureau, saw the governor's staff, and personnel of the Massachusetts Department of Public Health. In addition they sent a mimeographed letter to community residents as well as to members of the Center's policy committee and others urging their attendance at an open community meeting to protest the budget cut.

The meeting was chaired by Celia Holder, HAC's chairman, who did extremely well. Members of HAC turned out in full force as did more than 150 community residents. I had deliberately stayed clear of all their discussions and preparations and only at the last moment decided to attend the meeting—sitting in the back of the hall. Policy committee members called me several times before the meeting to ask how many people were expected, what the agenda was, and so on. I answered in perfect truth that I had no idea.

As the Boston *Herald Traveller* subsequently reported, some of Boston's top brass in health circles were present. I was particularly grateful that the director of the Radcliffe Institute, where I had spent so many pleasant hours, and a professor of social welfare at Brandeis, whose advice on community affairs I treasured, attended the meeting to give me personal support.

A number of commitments were made that night to the community, including HAC's right to screen potential candidates for my job, and subsequent to the meeting I got what I had long wanted: until I left the Center, eight members of HAC sat with the eight members of the policy committee to discuss health center policies. But the cuts were not restored, and I didn't rescind my resignation, though I was pleased that the policy committee, HAC, other community organizations, and Center staff asked me to change my mind. I had achieved my objectives. Professionals at health centers throughout the United States were enduring troubling confrontations with community boards, and many left their posts for this reason. I was fortunate that our community confrontation came about because residents valued *their* Center and supported me in my protest against the cuts we'd received.

On the other hand, Harry was pleased and relieved when I resigned. He was unhappy with the extent of my commitment to the job and worried about my safety when I went to those constant night meetings. But mainly he found my absorption in the Center's affairs hard to take. It was not that I neglected my family; the children and house remained chiefly my responsibility. But perhaps for a wife and mother of my generation my commitment and feelings of responsibility to the health center were too intense. Harry said there were times when he knew that though I listened, seemingly intently, when he spoke to me, my mind was miles away in Bracken Field. On one level he was right; I felt obligated to the community I had chosen to serve. But the benefit was not one-sided. Not since South African health center days had I felt the same deep satisfaction and fulfillment of making a difference to the lives of a neglected community.

At the farewell party the community gave me I laughed when I thought how shocked South African (and Bostonian) politicians would have been to see me dancing with black men. But I was sad to leave the people who meant so much to me, and I was moved by their speeches and their gifts. One of these, a painting, was presented by a black activist I knew. I'd been to his last exhibition and seen how he pictured his hostility to whites. As he came nearer with his package, I dreaded opening it, thinking how could I possibly hang such a picture on my walls. But when I uncovered the wrapping, I found a charming portrayal of a black family. While I was checking the files I still had on the health center, a month or so ago, I came across a faded copy of my letter of thanks. After all these years the memories it evoked still brought a lump to my throat. Because it is so very personal, I reproduce here only the last paragraph of that letter.

> But I will always remember my time with you and especially my last day as I remember that other day I told you of 15 years ago. And wherever I go I will take my gifts and my memories with me and it will be as if I have never left you.
>
> With deep affection
> Eva

When I finally left the Center, I spent a blissfully peaceful year as a Senior Associate at the Harvard Center for Community Health and Medical Care. During that year my colleagues and I wrote several articles reflecting the work of our research team.

As I mentioned earlier, we already knew from our household survey certain facts essential to the planning of our services, and some bear repeating as background information for the new information. Our area of service contained 6,000 children under the age of twenty-one and 2,000 women of child-bearing age; one-third of the children had only one parent in the home; and there was rampant geographic mobility. One-third of the households—whose residents were almost all black and who lived in the housing project—had 40 percent of the area's children, but in the total area to be served 61 percent of the households had white residents, 30 percent black, and 7 percent Hispanic. Twenty-nine percent of all families were on welfare, and a quarter of all the children of the area were less than five years old. The response to our center's presence was immediate and favorable: in the first twelve months of its operation 1,215 families registered for its services, and by the end of the second year 1,613 had done so.

Registration rates were highest in families who had the lowest

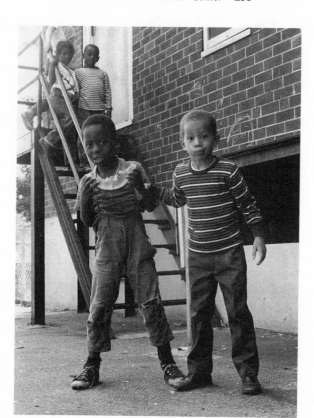

Bracken Field children

incomes, those who lived in the housing project, and those who received Aid to Families of Dependent Children—showing us that the families with the least access to conventional medical care were attracted to the health center at an exceptionally high rate. Indeed it was rumored that families with young children, and many problems, were given apartments in the housing project because of our being there.[6]

Our analysis of the care we had given to patients during 1968 showed that 87 percent had received at least one professional service; 70 percent of the children had been examined by a pediatrician; and most of the children had been seen by at least two different kinds of personnel, the commonest combination being pediatrician and dentist. Once families had decided to register, their race, place of residence, and family size and education had only a minor effect on their use of services at our center. Children's ages, however, markedly influenced their utilization rates—a greater proportion of preschool children than adolescents came for attention and attended more often. Since the children we looked after visited physicians and dentists far more frequently than the national norms for corresponding ethnic and socioeconomic groups, we concluded that the response to our health center had been most favorable and that the easy accessibility, reaching-out philosophy, and genuine concern of our staff had had a marked effect.[7]

Probing deeper, we selected a random sample of registered and unregistered households to ascertain residents' reactions and attitudes toward the institutions and professionals from whom they got their health care. We confirmed our previous finding that families who used the Center as their primary source of care were the ones who needed services the most. Those who used us expressed their satisfaction with the attitudes and attention of our staff. They were pleased with the convenience of the Center, its friendly and helpful atmosphere, ease in making appointments, shorter waiting periods and adequate time to spend with the doctors, who were thorough, kind, patient, and concerned. Of course they wanted much more from us—a twenty-four-hour facility which would completely replace the outpatient and emergency rooms of a hospital and yet remain a convenient neighborhood facility.[8]

Even today, Boston, with its unparalleled specialist resources and its extensive network of neighborhood health centers, has higher mortality rates for its black and low-income infants and young children.[9] Bracken Field showed me, once again, why diseases resulting from societal inequities can't be cured by medical care alone—no matter its excellence.

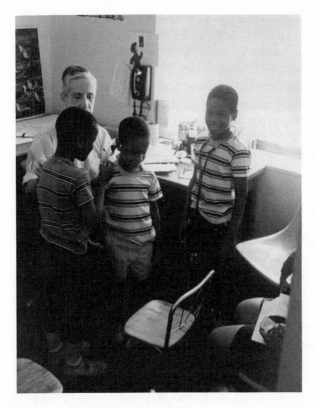

Children enjoying a visit to their doctor

But objective, epidemiologic data, essential as they are, only portray what can be measured. I was unhappy at confining research reports to what have been called defleshed statistics, and I wrote one rather passionate paper on the importance of community involvement in shaping neighborhood health center policies.[10] Yet I felt that even that kind of article was not enough and decided that only the people themselves could adequately describe their problems and emotions. I could draw them out, record their words, edit for others to read, but they, not I, must do the talking. So I began a series of unstructured, tape-recorded interviews with some of the people who either lived or worked in Bracken Field. Amy undertook the tiresome job of typing the original scripts verbatim and, later, the numerous edited versions which I mailed to her from Chapel Hill. It took five years from the time I began my first interview to the time the book was finally completed and published. Listening to these verbal accounts of people's lives, reading over and over again what they had told me, editing and reediting, was for me a necessary catharsis.[11]

Over the years, though I saw Bracken Field and its residents only seldom, I kept in touch. On one of my Boston visits I met Celia in her office at the Harvard Community Health Plan—a very large health maintenance organization. She'd finally realized her dream of buying a house outside Bracken Field, and she owned a car. Her walls were plastered with photographs: Celia with Kevin White, Celia with Ted Kennedy, etc. She seemed to be on every consumer committee in Boston and was very happy and self-confident. On another visit I introduced Arnold, an intern at the Brigham Hospital, whom I'd known as a Duke medical student. After questioning him thoroughly, Celia addressed him. "What did you say your name was, young man? I want you to know that I'm on the board of the Brigham Hospital, and I will keep an eye on your progress." Arnold was impressed. Not so Harry, when Celia told him the Massachusetts health commissioner's post was vacant, and if he wanted the job, she would put in a good word for him. Yet there were cracks in Celia's armor. She spoke better than she wrote and told me her biggest difficulty at work was learning to write memos. I assured her she would overcome that obstacle also.

The health center asked me to be their keynote speaker at their tenth anniversary dinner celebration—a joyous occasion. In March 1985 Celia, learning of my coming visit to Boston, instructed me to keep the Friday of that week for Bracken Field. She picked me up that morning and drove me to the project, which looked in much better physical shape than in my time and was now largely Hispanic. I was escorted through the Center by Mark Clay, Celia, and Stella Jones. They introduced me to the administrative director, who'd been there a record four years, and to the medical director who'd been there an astonishing nine years. It was obvious that the confrontational atmosphere of the sixties had vanished. The Center's administrative structure had been vastly simplified, all administration now coming directly under Children's Hospital. But to my great pleasure the overall aims of the health center were still the same as in 1967. The program had continued to expand: adult services were a feature and optometry had been added as a service. The Center was still heavily subsidized. The people it served remained the poor: 64 percent were on Medicaid, 12 percent had some type of health insurance, 24 percent had neither Medicaid nor private insurance and were unable to pay for their care. HAC had become the Community Advisory Board to Children's Hospital and had retained the rights it gained when I resigned.

A few employees from my time were still working at the Center. It was fun to see them, and I would have lingered longer had my escorts not hurried me to get to the luncheon which had been arranged. But at the last moment Stella whispered, "Wouldn't you like to see the medical records department? Molly's been our medical record librarian for ages, and she's doing a super job." We raced up the three flights of stairs and greeted Molly, who smiled with relief when she saw us. She thought we'd abandoned her. "I was just saying to myself that of course she won't come to see me. Of course, they won't bring her. I'm not important. I'm nothing to her. Nobody cares about me." Going down the stairs, I thanked Stella for her thoughtfulness, and I realized, once again, how fragile the new skin of confidence can be.

I was always drawn to Stella with her forthright speech, her defense of the underdog, her delight in shocking the prim and proper, her pugnacious stance hiding her soft heart. I smiled recalling some of her conversations with me:

"Dr. Salber, we're going to hold a meeting tonight to do something about the rats and roaches here. Something *has* to be done about them. We're talking about a rent strike. Maybe I'll sit in, in the Housing Office. Say Dr. Salber, if I sit in, would you see that I get plenty of beer?" (Stella subsequently deposited a dead rat in the Housing Office.)

"Dr. Salber, I've thought of a good way to get rid of roaches in Bracken Field. Frogs eat insects, so maybe they eat roaches. We could catch about 300 frogs and toads and let them loose in the project to eat the roaches."

"Dr. Salber, the nursery school teacher says my Derrick is doing fine now. He's just turned five. But some of the mothers are so damn stupid. One mother complained that Derrick was making love and doing wrong things to her daughter. What was he doing? Making movements with the lower part of his body to her. I said I was very pleased if Derrick was doing that to her daughter. It's a big step forward for him. Every time he used to see a girl, he used to fight her and pull her hair, so if he's making love to girls now that's a step in the right direction."

The afternoon of the party Stella herself displayed the fragile skin I'd witnessed in Molly. When she walked along with me after we left the luncheon, she told me how her sons had questioned her about what I was like. I waited: it's not often we get a frank assessment of ourselves, and Stella dealt hard punches. "I told them we'd all come and see you to complain about everything we didn't like, and we'd stand there and stamp our feet and shout, and you listened and never shouted back." And then she blurted out, "Dr. Salber, how can you spend the day with the likes of us?" We were walking past the Boston Public Library; the sidewalk and streets were crowded. We stopped in the middle of the crowd while I searched for healing words, but body language was better. I gave her a bear hug, and she understood, hugging me back.

The luncheon was in a private room of a downtown hotel, and we toasted each other in white wine. I didn't know all the seventeen people there, but it dawned on me that they were either present members of the Community Advisory Board or people I'd interviewed for my book. I asked the old-timers about their activities. Mark now worked for the Boston Housing Authority as Superintendent of Crime Prevention Community Affairs. He was also chairman of the Center's Community Advisory Board. His wife was now chairman of the Bracken Field Tenant Management Committee. The Bracken Field housing project was the first in Boston where a tenant group became responsible for the maintenance, care, and upgrading of the project. Mabel Straley, a longtime leader in community affairs, was executive director of the Tenant Management Group. Stella, a past Community Advisory Board member, was working as a licensed practical nurse in a home for the elderly and has now signed up for a gerontology course at a community college. Claude was director of communications in Bracken Field, responsible for the newsletter and the project's radio station, and a member of the management group. Mrs. Taylor had retired as an aide at the Center—she'd been working there from the time it first became a clinic—and was a "foster grandmother" in the oncology division of Children's Hospital. Celia had sixteen years to her credit at the Harvard Health Plan and was a member of the Bracken Field Community Advisory Board. One young woman at the lunch, vice-chairman of the Community Advisory Board, had been a pediatric patient when I was at the Center and now had six children of her own. She described herself to me as "poet, singer, performer, and good human being." The executive administrative director, medical director, and head nurse of the Center also attended the luncheon.

After a substantial lunch, much jollity, and taking of snapshots, Mark Clay made a short speech and then presented me with a handsome plaque. On it were the names of the six people at the lunch whom I had interviewed and who were still active in Bracken Field's affairs. It was a totally unexpected but joyous surprise. Mark read the inscription on the plaque.

This is a Token of Love
Presented to
Dr. Eva J. Salber

Who Taught Us that
Caring and Curing is a
Labor of Love and Respect

Mark Clay	Mrs. Taylor
Stella Jones	Celia Holder
Mabel Straley	Claude

1985

I was deeply touched, but for a moment I was also puzzled by the names Mark read out. I had been addressing my friends by their real names. They laughed at me. "Have you forgotten? We are using the names you gave us in the book."

Part Three. North Carolina

Samuel Johnson, or perhaps another, used to say

there was no man on the streets whose biography he would not like

to be acquainted with. No rudest mortal walking there who has not

seen and known experimentally something, which, could he tell it,

the wisest would hear willingly from him!

—Thomas Carlyle

Moving South: A New Beginning

Unexpectedly, one day in the spring of 1968 Harry was invited to consider a position as health commissioner to Cleveland, and I was promised a neighborhood health center job in that city. When he went for his second interview, I was asked to come as well.

I will never forget our meeting with Mayor Stokes. For at least an hour we debated frankly whether the mayor could employ a white South African as his health commissioner. We appreciated his dilemma, but for us the only reason for leaving Boston for Cleveland was precisely *because* we were white South Africans. Working for a black mayor might lessen the guilt we felt in running away from South Africa's racial problems. Finally, Mr. Stokes offered Harry the post believing that he was the right person for the job even though his background would be a hard pill for many blacks to swallow. He promised to send his letter of confirmation to our home in Newton.

But, a month or so later, a lengthy and regretful telegram replaced the expected letter. Mayor Stokes could not appoint Harry and knew we would understand his reasons without spelling them out explicitly. We did, perfectly, and though somewhat disappointed, we were also relieved. I'd been driven through a run-down area of the city to see the health center where I'd be working; it seemed a tough and scary neighborhood. And Harry wouldn't have considered Cleveland if not for Mr. Stokes. Cleveland was one of the cities where Martin Luther King's assassination touched off extended rioting—much of it in the area I would have worked in. Our position would have been impossible and a great burden on the mayor. At least we had made a gesture in the right direction, but racial prejudice is not confined to whites only.

Harry had become disheartened with the job he was in, and the Cleveland episode made him realize he didn't have to stay in Boston for the rest of his life. So he responded to a few attractive New York offers, but he found the city so oppressive that he never seriously considered moving there. The job he did decide to take turned out to be in Chapel Hill, North Carolina. Toward the end of the sixties, the federal government started a national program in health planning. Staff were needed for health planning councils (now known as health system agencies), and money was given to organizations like the University of North Carolina (UNC) School of Public Health at Chapel Hill to train personnel. Harry agreed to head that school's training program. He was ready to move on. I, on the other hand, was happily settled at Harvard's Center for Community Health and Medical Care and worried about the interruption of my community research.

But even aside from my work I was reluctant to move south in August 1970. Part of my disquiet came from my difficulty in uprooting myself from friends and familiar places, although I knew that this time I would be spared the feeling of isolation of my early Boston days because we already had some close expatriate friends in Chapel Hill. My deep disinclination to make the move stemmed rather from the fact that we had chosen to leave the "deepest South" when we left South Africa, and now we were choosing to return south to an analogous situation.[1]

This was 1970. It was only sixteen years after the Supreme Court ruling against segregated schools, ten years from the violence of the late 1950s and early 1960s, a mere five years since the implementation of the civil rights acts of the mid-1960s.

True enough North Carolina was not the deep south. Yet North Carolina has been called a paradox. While it was highly acclaimed for its support of higher education (largely a white monopoly), it ranked badly in elementary and secondary education. And though as early as the 1940s and 1960s North Carolina had a higher percentage of blacks registered and voting than any other southern state, by 1970 it stood last in this respect.[2]

Neither were the state's health statistics encouraging. In 1969–71 Massachusetts was placed fifteenth in the nation in longevity, but North Carolina only forty-fourth. In both these states whites lived longer than blacks, but the interstate differences were greater for blacks. In the mid-1960s the South had higher infant death rates for both whites and blacks than the Northeast—21.7 to 19.1 percent for whites and 40.5 to 33.8 percent for blacks. This excess in black infant deaths was largely due to the poverty and lower educational levels of minority groups. The same rationale can be applied to the higher death rates in nonmetropolitan than in metropolitan areas—particularly for black infants—and North Carolina was, and still is, a mainly rural state. But, regardless of region or residence, black babies in the United States as a whole had higher death rates than white babies.[3]

Nor, after spending so many years studying and trying to decrease smoking among young people, did I relish moving into a state so financially dependent on tobacco. But the work Harry was about to embark on was important, and I did not try to dissuade him.

When Massachusetts colleagues heard I was moving to a tobacco state, they were highly amused. But when I told the North Carolina Cancer Society I was preparing a paper on smoking in schoolchildren for an overseas conference and asked about their educational programs, they were *not* amused. There were other cancers than lung cancer, they said, asked why I needed to talk about smoking, and wanted to know how much publicity the conference would get. I tried the Heart Association next. This time I didn't say I was a doctor, or mention the conference, but merely requested information on the same material over the telephone. The answer came in a shocked voice, "Programs on smoking for schoolchildren? Lady, don't you know you're in a tobacco state?"

Harry had asked about a job for me and was assured that with two universities, UNC and Duke, within ten miles of each other,

I was sure to get a job. I was too busy the first few months in Chapel Hill to think about employment, since we were building a house and settling in, and I needed to get my bearings and find my way around—with my poor sense of direction always difficult for me in a new place. But when I did look for work, the right job was not simple to find, for the town spilled over with talented wives, much younger than I, whose husbands staffed the two universities.

One of the unexpected benefits of not having a job right away was that it gave me time to meet a remarkable group of "old-timey" blacks. Chapel Hill's small, black community lived in a cluster of streets close to the center of town in little, neatly kept houses with pocket-sized vegetable patches and brightly flowering gardens. The men were mostly artisans or laborers, the women domestics working for white families.

I'm not sure how I first saw Sarah Taylor, but when I did we felt an immediate kinship. When we met, she was still doing day work, and she came to clean for me too, but I often interrupted her chores with my questions. We always lunched together, but she wouldn't sit with us if Harry was there. I thought many times of interviewing her, on tape, and regret not having done so. Sarah often called me "Baby"—she must have been about fifteen years older than I was—and I told her she was my black mother.

Twice widowed, Sarah had only two surviving relatives: her daughter-in-law who taught school in Washington and her grandson, a boy of twelve when I met him spending his summer vacation with his grandmother. Sarah adored her grandson and willed her house to him. Her biggest wish was that he become a doctor, and I'm sad that I don't know whether he did. A tall, handsome dignified woman, Sarah was extremely intelligent, had a good sense of humor, and showed shrewd judgment. In another age she would have gone far, but orphaned as an infant and brought up by an aunt, she was taken out of school after the second grade. From the age of ten Sarah had labored in the cotton fields of South Carolina, as she put it, "from sunup to sundown and the sun riz early in South Carolina."

Sarah introduced me to Southern delicacies—pound cake, pecan pie, and chess pie, which I liked only too well, and collards, turnip greens, and okra which I didn't like at all. She also brought me cuttings from her flower garden and showed me how to use a pickax in our red clay soil. Sarah's white peonies still bloom in my garden to remind me of her each spring. She had lived in Chapel Hill for many years and had brought up the children of one family from infancy to marriage. When those children were grown, the family paid to have a house built for her. While I knew her, she built on an extra room because she had informally adopted a young lad whose mother had problems with alcohol. Harry and I were invited to the blessing ceremony for this room and the celebration lunch. The part-time minister of her church, a plasterer by trade, intoned the blessing. This was the first time—though by no means the last—that I witnessed a black congregation's responsiveness to its minister, a chorus of voices intoning "Go ahead . . . Uh huh . . . Praise the Lord . . . Yes, Preacher . . . Thank you Jesus . . . and Amen." As I looked and listened, I felt that their religion was not just a once-a-week, church-on-Sunday event. Sarah, too, had deep faith, but also a healthy scepticism toward a fellow churchwoman who "spoke with tongues."

When Sarah became ill with what later was diagnosed as an incurable cancer, I discovered firsthand the difficulties that the poor and uneducated face in getting services to suit their particular situations. She had excellent diagnostic "work-up," but at one stage the specialists decided she needed to be sent to a chronic care institution thirty miles from Chapel Hill. Her church and her friends were all in Chapel Hill, and she was despondent at the thought of living and dying among strangers. I told her I would do what I could to keep her home.

I won't spell out all the problems and indignities we went through in trying to get her a disability pension (which arrived after she had died). One illustration will suffice. Together we went to the welfare office sitting side-by-side facing the welfare worker who read aloud rapidly from a printed form. Sarah was astonished to be asked such questions as whether she owned a car and a boat and looked at me in bewilderment. When I told the worker that Sarah couldn't follow what was being read to her, "I'm required by law to read this to her" was her reply. At the end of the reading Sarah was told to sign her name. We both looked carefully at that form. To save money the welfare department was using up its out-of-date forms which, at that time, specified that a lien would be placed on the signer's house if a disability pension were granted. Sarah would sooner have been sent away herself than sign away her house. It took all my powers of persuasion, and her trust in my personal guarantee, to convince her that her house would not be taken after she was dead.

Sarah remained in Chapel Hill and continued to get her usual medical care at the local health center and the specialist clinics of the hospital. I arranged for a visiting nurse to look after her at home and hired someone from her church to spend several hours each day with her; church members and neighbors had already set up a rota of persons responsible for seeing to her meals. (She confided that the elderly man who made her breakfast was not a good cook—he scorched the grits.) I visited often and found her patient and stoic. But one day she was unusually depressed. Her doctor at the health center had told her there was no use her coming to see him again—there was nothing more he could do to make her better. I didn't say much to her but went home and appealed to the young man—whom I knew to be a kind and concerned individual—not to make Sarah lose all hope. Next day Sarah laughed as she asked, "What did you say to my doctor? He came to my house to see me!"

When I would tell people of the struggle to get Sarah homecare, they always responded, "She's lucky to have you." That remark irritated rather than pleased me, for I felt she should have been entitled to those services in her own right. Except for her last two days when she was admitted to the hospital because the intensity of her pain demanded constant medication, Sarah remained at home in moderate comfort with her good friends in attendance. She was eulogized in her church—I was asked to say a few words too—but I saw with sadness at the funeral that she was far more expensively dressed in death than she had been in life. Her family motioned me to sit beside them in church and invited me to ride with them to the burial service. I was grateful because I had long thought of Sarah as part of my family.

Through Sarah I met many other old-timers. They were solid citizens of deep faith, uncomplaining about hard work for modest pay, caring for their neighbors, enjoying good company, and relishing a hearty laugh. They made me feel a part of Chapel Hill—no longer a stranger to the South. And often their kindness in service to others, their sense of fun—and their color—reminded me of Sakkie and my youth.

Estelle, who came to help me after Sarah died, was the aunt of a colleague and became a dear friend. We solved the name problem quickly. When she called me "Ma'am," I called her "Mrs. Gattis"; when she called me "Eva," I called her "Estelle"; when her niece and I talked about her we both called her "Aunty." And when our house is about to receive a deluge of visitors, or children and grandchildren, Estelle comes to my aid, and we spend a busy day in the kitchen—her pound cakes are in the same class as Sarah's.

It was Estelle who referred a neighbor, Mr. Edwards, to me as an occasional, garden/outdoor worker. He listened to my requirements in silence before he said, "Ma'am, I have to tell you. I had a lot of accidents when I worked. I got only one good arm, I got a knee-cap gone on one leg, my back been fused. But I reckon, if I takes my time, I can help you!"

I marvel at Mr. Edwards' pluck and stamina. He has a sunny nature and enjoys the amusement he gets from his fellowmen. Harry has a very companionable relationship with him; Edwards often shakes his head, laughs, and tells me, "I declare! That man tickles me." Harry says I must be the only person in Chapel Hill to greet Edwards formally as "Mr. Edwards." Another man, whom I also address formally as Mr. MacDuffie, is a house-painter, carpenter, electrician, a real handyman. I asked Mr. Edwards one day if he knew Mr. MacDuffie and was most surprised when he said he didn't. MacDuffie, in turn, denied knowing Edwards. Since the older black community in Chapel Hill is so small and stable, I couldn't understand how this was possible. One day both men happened to be at our house at the same time and greeted each other warmly. Somewhat miffed, I demanded to know, "Why did you both tell me you didn't know each other?" MacDuffie answered, "I never heard anyone call him by the name you said—everyone round here calls him "Pop," and they call me "T.J."

At the same time as I was beginning to know Chapel Hill's black community, I was also learning about innovative student activities in caring for some of the poor citizens of Durham. A week after we moved to Chapel Hill, I met John, a UNC medical student who was working in a "free clinic" in a run-down area of Durham. This Edgemont clinic, housed in a ramshackle dwelling in a mixed neighborhood, operated surprisingly well considering its chronic state of bankruptcy. Most of its help came from UNC's teaching hospital, which provided supplies and preceptors for the students. Students raised what money they could and employed two part-time neighborhood aides and a part-time receptionist/record-keeper. John and a fellow student were members of the clinic board chaired by a woman of the area well known for her devotion to this and other community projects. A few other women residents, both black and white, completed board membership. Because John had visions of turning the clinic into a neighborhood health center, he asked for my help, and I went with him to the evening clinics and sat in on board meetings held in a tiny attic room. So pressing was the lack of funds that I brought my own chair to the meetings and left it there. I was invited to join their board, and I tried very hard to increase financial support for the clinic.

I failed miserably in persuading two men, prominent in medical education at the two universities, that the clinic was an important educational tool. The Duke professor was regarded as conservative, his UNC equivalent as liberal and forward-looking in health affairs, yet they had the same attitude to the clinic. Without spending time there, both felt that the quality of care given by the students and their preceptors was inferior and should not be supported. They didn't see benefits for the patients. What surprised me much more was their not recognizing the benefit of this exposure to the needs of a poor community for the students themselves.

I was surprised, also, to learn how many hospital physicians were oriented to institutions and not to communities. When they talked about community, they meant doctors who practiced outside the hospital setting, not the patients. When I suggested that medical students at Duke should follow some of the patients they saw in the hospital into those patients' homes, the answer I got shook me. "Who," I was asked, "would pay for their transportation and their insurance?"

Fortunately, the students at the clinic were not easily discouraged. One severe winter, having run out of wood, they kept a fire in the grate to warm the place by burning linoleum torn from the floor! Without funds and with little university support the clinic finally closed in 1978. But a year later with new support, students opened another free clinic in a different area of Durham—its philosophy clearly stated in a flyer announcing the opening. "The East End Health Center is run by the people of the East End. The Center should be a center for the people, by the people, and of the people of the East End."

My first real chance of a job I wanted to do came through the good offices of Dr. Harvey Estes, chairman of the Department of Community and Family Medicine at Duke Medical School. A kind, gentle, and extremely modest physician, Estes arranged a meeting for me with Charles Watts, a prominent black surgeon, who was trying to convert Lincoln Hospital—Durham's black community hospital—into a neighborhood health center. In the United States if a hospital or a school was named Lincoln, it was almost certain to be black.

I thought a lot about Lincoln Hospital in the week before my appointment with Dr. Watts. Lincoln Hospital was old; built not only to accommodate black patients during a time of segregation, but also to provide residency training posts for black doctors. Because I can lose my way even in a one-way street, I carefully wrote Dr. Watts' directions to Lincoln Hospital on an index card and did a trial run the day before my appointment. I was reminded of the period in Boston when I worked with twenty-seven hospitals and carried in my pocketbook twenty-seven cards; one side had directions to each hospital, and the other instructions for getting back to home base. I was too embarrassed to ask Dr. Watts for directions to get back home and was afraid that if I did ask he would think me too stupid to employ, but after the trial run I wrote down the return route also.

Charles Watts was an impressive man—highly intelligent, good-humored, and open. He consistently breached the color bar: as the first black doctor in the medical society, the first black member of Durham's Chamber of Commerce, the first black chairman of the Health System Agency. His interest in getting a neighborhood health center was not really a wish to change the way medicine was practiced, but rather a means to save Lincoln Hospital from closing down and to increase the small number of black doctors and dentists in Durham.

Prior to the passage of Medicare and Medicaid legislation in the mid-sixties, Durham's white community hospital, (coincidentally named Watts Hospital) hadn't admitted black patients, but after this legislation and consequent integration of patients it began to draw patients away from Lincoln Hospital. Duke University Hospital had admitted blacks from the time it opened in the thirties. Ironically, because of integration, Lincoln Hospital, while still regarded with much pride, was no longer essential to the black community, and its beds were underused. The hospital was steadily losing money. So Dr. Watts was negotiating with the federal government for money to convert the hospital's ambulatory department into a neighborhood health center, had gotten a small grant for his program, and had hired a competent administrative secretary. At the end of our meeting he asked if I would be willing to help him as a consultant and wanted to know how much time I could give to the project. I had just begun editing drafts of interviews for my book on the Bracken Field Health Center, but I promised two days a week and hoped I could stick to that schedule.

Almost immediately I began my work and was paid for two days a week, but I was so engrossed and there was so much to do that I found myself going to work each day, attending meetings at night, and working full-time as the second staff person rather than as a part-time consultant. Dr. Watts gave me a desk in his office, and we were soon on a first name basis. He seemed equally at home in Lincoln's shabby office as he was in his sumptuous office at the North Carolina Mutual Life Insurance Company—the largest black insurance company in the world—where he was the medical director. Charles Watts drove to work in his white Cadillac (which he changed each year for a new model), and I in my small Fiat. He was the first black person I met who was prepared to share ethnic jokes with me, being comfortable enough to use the term "nigger" when that was part of the story. I reciprocated with typical, self-deprecatory Jewish jokes.

Though I was familiar with black poverty, this was my first entry into a black middle-class world. Charlie and his family lived in a house near the hospital, but many well-to-do black professionals, businessmen, and educators lived in a secluded enclave of Durham that resembled white suburbia right down to the requisite country club.[4] I visited the area and found the tenor distinctly conservative—light years removed from the Bracken Field housing project. Even Charlie, who was looked up to by poor and wealthy alike, was far more class-conscious than I was. Once when we returned from a community meeting, where I had thought him to be rather high-handed and dogmatic, I took him to task. "If I had spoken to those people the way you did, they'd have called me a white racist pig. You can get away with it because you're a black man." Charlie was not the least bit fazed, but often thereafter called me his "community teacher."

Gradually we acquired an entirely female staff to head departments of nursing, social work, medical records, and so on and, at the beginning, an exclusively male staff of doctors and dentists. Female staff would often voice their dissatisfactions to me but would never complain openly to Dr. Watts. At staff meetings I would encourage them, egg them on. "Come on sisters, tell him now." They never did. It was a time when black women believed they should hold themselves back and push their men forward.

The most assertive men I met were those who were politically ambitious, heading for positions in local or state government. But, in general, southern blacks were not assertive, showing more gentleness and friendliness than their northern brothers. The passivity of the Lincoln Advisory Board was in marked contrast to most such boards in Boston. This submissive behavior certainly made the lives of professional staff much easier—my own included—and no one besides myself seemed to feel a need to educate the board members to play a more active role.

White southerners were also less aggressive, ambitious, and sophisticated than northerners and were friendly and easy to get along with. But many still had a strong dislike for liberal Yankees, particularly those from New York. Some men I knew gloated when New York City was close to bankruptcy in the mid-1970s. As the wave of northerners retiring to Chapel Hill swelled, I heard irritation toward New Yorkers expressed. "Too many people from Wesschess [Westchester] here." A North Carolina senator is reported to have said it was not necessary for the state to build a zoo; all that was needed was to put a fence around Chapel Hill.

As we built up our staff at Lincoln and prepared for clinical services, I worried about the smallness of the center's budget and prepared a more realistic one. Charlie agreed that the new budget should be presented to the regional headquarters of the U.S. Government's Department of Health, Education, and Welfare (DHEW) in Atlanta and asked me to accompany him there. Since our appointment was in the early morning, we needed overnight accommodation, but Charlie seemed dissatisfied with the only available choice. Arriving at the Atlanta airport in the late evening in the rain, he rented a car and drove to this motel. I was left in the car—ostensibly to stay dry—while he confirmed our reservations. Tackled at breakfast, Charlie admitted his fear that we'd have been refused accommodation had we gone in together. I was reminded of the time when I asked a Lincoln board member, who was also a professor of health education, whether he liked movies. He told me he'd seen very few, since cinemas had been segregated until recently. Black friends also told me that, not too many years back, vacations meant going to visit relatives, since motels wouldn't accept them—their journey made worse by the lack of toilet facilities on the way. South Africa seemed near at hand. I recalled the market square in the small South African town where we had spent the night in our car, defiantly and uncomfortably, because Katy, our colored nanny, had been refused a room at our hotel.

Charlie and I had a highly successful meeting in Atlanta and left feeling very pleased with ourselves. On the way back to the airport he gave me a tour of Atlanta—his hometown. He showed me the area where he'd sold newspapers as a boy, the college he'd attended, the Ebenezer Church, Martin Luther King's grave, the prosperous-looking section of Atlanta where middle-class blacks lived. Very proudly Charlie pointed out Atlanta's black insurance company—the *second* largest in the United States.

DHEW gave us the money we requested, and Charlie asked me to become the director of the Lincoln Community Health Center. It was exactly the job I wanted to do, and I rushed home to tell Harry the good news. But it made Harry very unhappy. He worried that I'd get involved in another controversial, difficult situation and said he wanted to protect me from myself. I'd be struggling with the same problems as in Bracken Field, and I'd be going back nights to meetings all the time. He couldn't face another period like the Bracken Field one, and he begged me not to take the job. I understood his feelings and knew that he read me right. I would inevitably become as absorbed in the Lincoln Center as I had been in the Bracken Field Center, but the direction of my life had led me to love and care for my family *and* to respond to the needs of a neglected community. How does one resolve the conflict between loyalty to family and to community? I didn't take the job, and I was depressed. I felt that I was nothing but a middle-class housewife of no use to anyone outside the family.

I wrote to Amy (my friend and secretary at the Bracken Field Health Center) and told her it seemed one simply *had* to have a job in order not to be lonely in a university town. I shared with her my thoughts about what I might do. In my fantasies I wanted to do more for the Edgemont Clinic, change health care in Durham, make an impact on the universities, etc., but these were only dreams, for I learned that foundations wouldn't give me support for Edgemont unless I had a faculty appointment and that this fact applied also to the book I was trying to write. My spirits were at a low ebb. It was not my year. Nor my town.

I remained at Lincoln part-time until a director was appointed and soon after that gave a dinner party in her honor inviting board members, staff, and spouses. One ambitious young husband of a black staff member, who was beginning his ascendancy in local politics, told the assembled group that he had no time for liberals. In fact he preferred dealing with right-wing conservatives like Ellis (a former Klansman) because you knew exactly where you stood with them and you never knew where you really stood with liberals.

South African blacks often felt the same way. When the Afrikaner Nationalist government came to power in 1948, many blacks said they preferred the Boer, "who would hate nakedly," to the "hypocritical English [who] . . . smiled at you with their front teeth and chewed you with their back teeth."[5]

I'd heard such sentiments often enough in Boston, too, and didn't take them personally, but Charlie was shocked and rushed to my defense. "When did you have dinner in Ellis's house?" he demanded to know. "We are having dinner in Eva's house. When we say 'You all' we don't include Eva." Others echoed his feelings, wrapping me in their friendship. My spirits lifted, and my depression melted.

I thought again of Dr. Estes and his department, so different in its philosophy from the rest of Duke medical school. He had understood my needs and had steered me to Lincoln. Perhaps he could find me another community to work in, less demanding of my time, but where I could feel equally useful. I would call for an appointment.

Settling Down at Duke

In 1971, after I left the Lincoln Community Health Center, I returned to academia—to Dr. Estes's Department of Community and Family Medicine at Duke University, where I stayed until I retired in 1982. In America, generally, departments of community and family medicine don't get the appreciation they deserve, and Duke was no exception. I feel such departments should be the basic clinical and teaching departments of medical schools because they focus on primary care to families and communities. In contrast, Duke's prestigious medical school emphasized the individual patient, professional specialization, and high technology.

I was happy, however, in the department of my choice, devoting my energies to community research, teaching, and action. I had the freedom—provided I could get the necessary funding, a recurrent anxiety—to do research on social, economic, and environmental issues, to explore how the medical care system responded to a community's requirements, to design programs to meet these needs, and to involve medical students in community health care. And I was free to report my findings in human as well as in statistical terms. This opportunity was of vital importance to me, making it possible to pass on to students the feelings of the men and women with whom I worked as "people of flesh and blood, who laugh and cry, who love and hate, who enjoy being cuddled." [1]

In one of my early jobs in the department, I became a consultant to the area Health Planning Council. For some years there had been a move to build a racially integrated hospital to replace black Lincoln Hospital and white Watts Hospital, and my assignment was to consider the future functions of these two hospitals after the new one was built. My suggestion was to develop the plan in the broader context of health care needs for all of Durham County's residents.

Health Planning Council staff and I brought together a hundred interested Durham residents, grouped these volunteers into committees, and for nine months studied all aspects of community health. Together we brought out a report and most of our recommendations—expansion of primary care centers, encouragement of group practice, the use of auxiliary medical and dental workers, expanded health education of the public— were accepted for implementation.[2] There were of course a few dissenters who thought my ideas too radical. One man balked at my suggestion that low-income housing in rural areas be expanded and upgraded. "What's that got to do with health?" he asked sarcastically. Another questioned my emphasis on broad community representation. "I suppose you'd like to have a five-year-old boy and a felon on your board," he grumbled. But almost everyone was forward-looking, agreeable, enthusiastic, and hardworking. For me, that planning project was an extraordinary opportunity to learn about the complex network of health-related agencies servicing the county and stood me in good stead in later work.

But my long-term, special satisfaction came from detailed studies of a smaller, rural area, beginning with a health interview survey in Bragtown and the adjoining villages of Rougemont and Bahama. Bragtown, with about 5000 residents living in 1200 households, was 80 percent black and contained three low-income housing projects and many young children. Rougemont/ Bahama, with about 2000 persons living in 700 households, was 80 percent white. Fortunately, I had access to an old friend, who was a national expert in survey research. He predicted—and proved to be right—how many interviews we could expect each interviewer to complete each day and why we could anticipate more than a 90 percent response rate in our, as yet, undersurveyed rural area. Thinking of that time brings to mind a cartoon

I cherished in oversurveyed Boston. It showed a student with clipboard and pencil, looking at a black woman standing in her doorway, arms akimbo, who is saying plaintively, "Well, are you from Harvard, Tufts, or B.U.?"

In our survey we wanted to know people's ages, the work they did, the illnesses they'd been through, the barriers they faced in getting care, whom they went to, what it cost them, what medications they took, whether their age, race, sex, and income affected the care they got, and other like questions. Preparing the detailed questionnaire took a long time, but mapping the areas and locating every house (many hidden from casual view at the end of narrow dirt roads) was even more trying. Often the most difficult problem was finding out in advance the race of householders; blacks would accept white interviewers, but the reverse was not as true, particularly in the rural area.

My staff scoured the area to get the names and race of householders. They drove, walked, talked to ministers, health advisory board members,[3] and even to the men who read the electricity meters. Discreet inquiries to residents about other people who lived on their road also helped, and cordial relations with postmasters proved invaluable.

One of our white interviewers, the wife of a Duke professor, found herself interrogating her own black garbage man. To Frances's surprise she found him to be a happy man secure in the knowledge that he, like his father and his aunt, was a member of an old established family of importance to the community. I thought of Sarah Taylor. If she had been in our survey, she, also, would have been placed in the lowest occupational category of unskilled worker. Statistical science deals with the collection and analysis of facts that can be stated numerically; surveys don't take community esteem into account.

Every interviewer met elderly persons who were lonely and pleased to have them visit, and all were asked for advice on medical, social, and economic problems. We always tried to help—through referral to medical care for those with no regular doctor, through information on how to go about getting food stamps, Supplemental Security Income, or legal aid—and we told everyone that Lincoln health center had opened a satellite clinic in Bragtown and in Rougemont/Bahama. While most residents were happy to learn of this conveniently placed facility and its transportation pickup service, some said they wouldn't have anything to do with "that clinic for folks who just laid on their backs and refused to work," and a few even sneered at "that nigger clinic."

Carolyn's field assignment included one rural segment which turned out to be a heavily patronized drinking area. Fortunately, she had been shown the correct way to leave a house so its residents wouldn't suspect her of being in cahoots with revenue agents![4] We'd warned field staff not to do evening work without an escort, but Carolyn usually ignored our warnings and found adventures in daytime as well as in evening hours. One day, entering a house "way in the sticks," Carolyn found a woman washing an enormous red spot on an older man's hip and was told that the man had been set on fire one midnight in revenge for an earlier killing. He was burned from armpit to knee and had gotten skin grafts in the hospital. Tisha, whose interviewing area bordered on Carolyn's, commented that several residents spoke of their neighbors as "bootleggers," but she was more troubled when they referred to her as a "carpetbagger."

We followed up our first survey with four additional visits to all the rural homes, concentrating on the illnesses each household member suffered and what actions they took. Some people got tired of being asked the same questions about their ailments so many times, yet we had very few refusals—most uncompleted interviews resulted from people moving out of the area to look for better jobs. But we must have tried people's patience sorely for we seldom took no for an answer. When an interviewer reported that her client seemed less cooperative than usual, we sent Becky, our most experienced and skilled interviewer. When all else failed, I telephoned the householders and apologized for our disturbing them. Some were so taken aback by these calls that they agreed to yet another interview—though I always felt a twinge of guilt at the power "Doctor" gave me.

Although we had a few disagreeable incidents, kindness and cooperation were the rule. I found these rural people to be gentler, less suspicious, and easier to interview than urban Boston residents. Often we were invited to meals, given freshly picked vegetables, and asked to come back. Whenever I came home laden with corn and tomatoes, Harry would laugh and say, "I thought you went to work today."

Our fieldwork took place over a three-year period, and we learned a great deal—enough to fill ten articles and three doctoral dissertations, but I'll limit reporting the findings of this study to a few sentences here. We found a strikingly low use of physician and dental services compared with the nation as a whole, particularly on the part of the black population, the poor, and the elderly. Rural black people very seldom went to private doctors. Those who were black, poor, elderly, *and* rural got the least attention of all.

We suggested these findings might be due to the brief interval since racial integration of services, the fact that no primary-care doctor practiced in this rural area, and the reluctance of Durham County's white doctors to accept Medicaid patients. We were seeing a community in a state of transition from the preintegration period, with its inequality of access to medical and dental services, to postintegration, with its freer access for all persons. Although much improvement had occurred in employment, income, and social mobility of blacks, established patterns of medical practice behavior were slower to change.[5]

After learning how two particular communities used medical services, we began to look at the profession responsible for providing these services. We analyzed the primary health care system in all of Durham County using data from all the medical institutions and almost 100 percent of private physician practices. We wanted to be able to answer the question: Who gives care to whom?[6] Though what we found was not unexpected, it still frustrated and depressed me. Access to health care was grossly unequal. The majority of white patients, most of whom had private health insurance, were looked after by specialists in private practice, but the majority of black patients, who seldom had private insurance, were seen mainly at Duke's public outpatient clinics, the Lincoln Community Health Center, and the Durham County Health Department. And we saw again, in this expanded canvas, what we'd learned in our earlier analysis of a section of the county—removal of legal and financial barriers had made little difference to the patterns of health care delivery which had been there before mandatory racial integration of health services.

Duke University's teaching hospital was so large, prestigious, and influential that while we'd included it in this overall investigation, we also studied it in more detail by itself. Duke Hospital has both a private diagnostic clinic and a public out-patient clinic system—modeled after the usual American teaching hospital of the time. Not surprisingly, we found that patients attending the private clinic for primary care were predominantly white and covered by private insurance, while those who went to the public clinics were largely black and heavily dependent on Medicaid coverage. We had no definitive data on the effect of different settings and clientele on the quality of medical education and patient care, but we assumed that sensitive teaching and excellent care would be far more difficult to get in the out-patient section of a two-class system of care.[7]

The article we wrote did not endear us to some members of the Duke establishment. A high-ranking administrator even questioned the validity of our data. I was reminded then of a previous time when I got into hot water with some of Harvard's top people. I'd returned from vacation to find that medical students had included me in a panel, scheduled for the following day, to fight Harvard's plan of combining several of its hospitals into one very large structure and demolishing low-rental apartments in the process. I was teamed up with a tenant representative and Mel King, a prominent black activist of Boston's South End, to oppose the overall designer of the plan, the dean of the medical school, and the heads of Harvard's teaching hospitals. As I took my place, plucked up my courage, and gave my views about people being more important than buildings, I saw the looks of disapproval on those professorial faces. "This is not the road to academic promotion," I said to myself. "You've really ditched it this time."

As the meeting ended, a Harvard professor I knew socially came up to me. "You spoke very well," he told me, "but Dr. X—— will never forgive you." In the split second in which memory traverses time, I saw the Sir Henry Elliott hospital in Umtata, South Africa, and heard its director's voice admonishing me. I'd been telling him about the house Harry and I would have one day and describing how my study would have bookshelves from floor to ceiling. "You'll never have a house, Dr. Salber," he told me. "You'll never have your own study. You'll just go from one poorly paid job to another."

Fortunately, there were other voices to listen to. My work in the Community Health Models unit was not confined to research, for I was also a teacher to a remarkable group of Duke medical students. They gave me a sense of identity, apart from that of wife and mother, a recognition of my individuality that warmed and strengthened me. Teaching was a giving and a receiving, a way to remember and to be remembered.

Before coming to Duke I'd done a lot of teaching: in Durban I taught doctors and nurses and health assistants in training at the Institute of Family and Community Health; at the Harvard School of Public Health, as a full-time researcher, I gave many lectures on the studies I was engaged in, most often at large meetings; and at the Bracken Field Health Center I was caught up with the education of the residents we served. But in the Department of Community and Family Medicine I indulged in the intimate teaching I enjoyed most—working intensively with a few students at each course offering.

Most Duke students were headed for a career in academic teaching, research, or private clinical practice as specialists and subspecialists. Very few were interested in primary health care, still less in care directed at whole communities instead of the individual patient. Once, after I'd given a formal lecture to a class of medical students, two immediately belittled my ideas. The first asked, "Why would a physician go into an unscientific area like community health sciences rather than a scientific discipline like internal medicine or surgery?" The second questioned the role of consumers in health planning and referred to them, only half in jest, as pollutants!

In contrast, I felt connected to my special young students, to whom I could pass on my beliefs about the responsibilities of physicians, my feelings about the people I served, and my values. The common factor uniting these students was what Chekhov called a talent for humanity.

A colorful and diverse lot, one was an artist, another a scholar in French, a third a marathon runner of near Olympic stature, a fourth (the son of an oil executive) a former college dropout. Several of the women were ardent feminists, in a group that included Jews, Catholics, agnostics, and Protestants of various denominations, including born-again Christians. One of the women had tried, unsuccessfully, to convert to Judaism because her socially conscious high school friends had all been Jews; another, whom I thought to be Jewish because she wanted to work in Israel, turned out to be a Baptist. Most had well-heeled parents, but none showed off their wealth in dress or manner. All were bright, vivacious young people possessed of enormous energy, eager to make the world a better place. I often wondered when they slept.

Why was I so taken with these young men and women? Partly because they were looking for a role model, and some used me that way, partly because we shared the same ideals of service to communities and partly—where I was certainly no role model—because they were physically so much braver than I.

Every time I drove alone at night to community meetings far from home, I gritted my teeth—I was so afraid of losing my way and spending the night marooned in my car on some unknown dirt road. Yet my student, Chris, organized her own field trip to four women's health collectives—in Chicago, Iowa City, Chico, and Los Angeles—by responding to an advertisement and driving someone's car from Durham to Los Angeles. Nancy worked with a group of black teenagers and won their respect when she took part in a grueling outdoor exercise—including swinging by rope from one tree to another—got hurt in the process and refused to give up. Diana taught Hmong refugees in Seattle and later as a pediatric resident looked after Hmong mothers and children in a camp on the northern Thailand-Laos border. Alan spent a summer in a clinic in Uganda during a time of bloody unrest. Marcia used her summers as an undergraduate to work in turbulent Latin American countries. And those who focused on the United States worked in our *own* Third World.

Women students had the additional burden of being female in a field still dominated by males. Another Nancy (names tend to have popularity cycles), whose fieldwork was with migrant farm workers, was chosen as student representative at a dinner honoring a well-known British physician. Seated next to the physician's wife—herself a doctor—she was told by her that married women should give up their professions and get their fulfillment from their husbands and children. Next morning she came to my office, fuming. "Doesn't she understand that we want both? She should encourage us, not make us feel guilty. Some women manage to do both. How did *you* do it?" We spent the next hour talking about the difficulties of combining motherhood and medicine and the practical kind of help which makes it possible.

Of all my students I know Marcia best; unlike the others, she remained in the area, and we regarded her as a surrogate daughter. As a medical student, she fretted that her regular courses were not related to the needs of poor communities and worried where she'd fit in as a doctor. So she joined the North Carolina Student Rural Health Coalition—representing medical, nursing, public health, law, and humanities students of several North Carolina universities—which promoted rural health by means of summer health and food fairs and designed a training curriculum for its organizers. As a married woman, she found her residency period in family practice almost inhuman in its demands—a common experience, especially for women graduates, and not confined to family practice. When her son was born, she had already accepted a fellowship in Preventive Medicine and for twelve months expressed her breast milk—kept in bottles in her freezer—so her son would not be deprived.

But no matter how independent and feminist these women were, they needed the nourishment of approval from someone with whom they could share their thoughts and feelings, and I needed their friendship and approval just as much. I still treasure Nancy's letter thanking me "for being interested in me, for caring about teaching me, and for encouraging me to care about others."

All my students were activists: organizing and staffing free clinics, setting up health fairs, tutoring backward children, teaching sex education in the schools, volunteering in the North Carolina Hunger Coalition, exposing the unconscionable conditions of migrant farm laborers, arranging seminars for fellow students, and publicizing their indignation at the poverty and lack of care they saw. They made me feel that Virchow's dream of doctors being attorneys for the poor might somehow, someday, yet be realized. Larry is a good example of how they all used our shared values in giving service to others—I have his reports and will quote him freely.

Larry served as an editor on *First Contact*, the Duke medical school student publication on primary care. I assigned him a difficult task: to assess the health of adolescents living in Warren County, one of the poorest counties in North Carolina.

The flavor of his report is apparent in his opening paragraph. "At a quick glance Warren is one more desolate 'food and fuel' along the interstate between Richmond and Raleigh, a series of crumbling whistle-stops along the Seaboard tracks. . . . The land grew cotton until it wore out, then new laws and new machines took the crop South to big scale farming. In Warren tobacco took over, setting the style and pace of life in the county."

Larry traced the history of the county and interviewed more than twenty of its community leaders. I still have the book he gave me describing the unwilling migration north of thousands of rural, black youth on buses or trains like the Chickenbone Special,[8]—the name comes from the fried chicken lunches mothers gave their children for the journey.

Shortly before his graduation Larry made me an unusual offer. He'd earned all the credits he needed to graduate, had a month to spare, and would willingly volunteer his time if I needed him. I'd been meeting with a county health director who was concerned about the dreadful environmental conditions in one of his small communities. When he asked for my help in developing a community health education program to go along with his environmental plan, I sent Larry to survey the area.

Northern Fairview was at the time an unincorporated area and therefore lacking in services. As Larry described it later, it contained "some 200 small, frame houses clustered together in various states of disrepair. Nearly a quarter of the homes lacked toilets and almost as many lacked running water. The soil was unsuited to outhouses and septic tanks, and house lots were criss-crossed with trickles of raw sewage seeping into wells and lying stagnant in ditches at the side of the dirt roads." (Northern Fairview was a black bedroom community; most of its inhabitants worked at the two universities—Duke and UNC.)

Today the area has piped water and a good sewerage system thanks to the Health Department, the county Planning Department, the efforts of many good citizens, and some federal support. But Larry's memories were of Northern Fairview as he'd seen it first, and together with Warren County they had a marked effect on him. As editor of the medical student periodical, he wrote, "Until medical students see the outhouses and sewage, until they listen to a single mother raising her family on $4000 a year, they are doomed to become another generation of burned-out-do-gooders full of prejudice and paternalism. In the interest of good medicine, it is time for the university, in teaching and example, to show students what life is like outside the doors of the hospital."

It was while I was revising this chapter that, quite by accident, I felt a lump in my belly and was catapulted into the lap of a large teaching hospital. I learned, very quickly, about the marvels of modern medical technology: ultra sound, CT-scans, anesthesia, and major abdominal surgery. I learned, also, that my dignity as a doctor was of small account once I put on the ridiculous hospital gown all patients must wear, which exposed my bare bottom when I walked in the hospital corridors. I learned how much better care married people get than single persons—spouses can act as special duty nurses and as patient advocates in addition to the comfort and support of their presence. And I learned that sensitivity to patients' needs seems insufficiently stressed in the curriculum of today's medical students.

On the afternoon of my admission I was firmly connected to a needle in my left arm from which a long tube led to a bag of intravenous fluid hanging from a large pole. I couldn't go anywhere, including the bathroom, without pushing that pole in front of me. That was a nuisance, but the "bowel prep" was a horror. My personal physician was on vacation, and no one had explained the details. Around seven that evening a gallon jar of GoLitely—a devilishly ironic name—was brought in, and I was instructed to drink it over the next four hours to clean out my system. Each succeeding cup of the liquid quickened my pace to the bathroom. Sometime between nine and ten that night a third-year medical student I'll call Peter—doing his surgery rotation—appeared in my room, informed me I was his patient, and told me he'd come to take my history and examine me. Since I believe it's grossly unfair for only the poor to be used as teaching material, I didn't send him away, but I expressed strong doubts on how it could be done. For the next hour and a half my answers to Peter's questions were increasingly interrupted by "Excuse me," as my pole and I ran. But, undaunted, Peter continued the examination, even to the extent of looking in my ears. When I finally thought I was rid of him, he suddenly reappeared. "I forgot to feel your thyroid," he said. Then the night nurse took over her end of the prep and at three, on the morning of my operation, I fell asleep for a couple of hours. I'm hazy about the exact time, but I think it was around six that Peter reappeared. "I forgot to ask you about your childhood illnesses," he announced.

A couple of days after my operation when "the team" of chief surgical resident, senior and junior residents, and four third-year medical students did their rounds, I parodied Peter's encounters with me and told them I'd pay my hospital bill by sending a script to Woody Allen. The chief resident said that Peter was "a driven student." "Yes," I replied, "but who drives him?" The teacher in me would not be denied as I read them a lecture: medical students must be taught, repeatedly and by example, that the patient is first and foremost a person, and there are times when examining a patient should be postponed.

It was then I recognized fully that I was writing my book as a teacher reaching out to unknown students and doctors—asking them to remember the people I was describing who needed their understanding and compassion as much as their technical knowledge. And, as I drifted into sleep that night—with the aid of a pill called *Halcion*—I thought how lucky I had been to have worked with so many dedicated students who would never need to be reminded.

Health Facilitators: Lay Advisers in Community Health

Some time back a letter came to me from Savu Savu, Fiji. "Dear Dr. Salber," it began, "Bula! Greetings from the South Seas! In a neighbor's home here in Fiji during a recent hurricane, I chanced upon an old "Mother Earth News" article written about your work. . . ."

That article had been reprinted from an issue of "Medical Self Care" in which the editor interviewed me,[1] and it prompted many people to write to me. Before Savu Savu the most unusual address had been the *Rainbow Warrior* Greenpeace ship and before that a local women's prison. The correspondents were often nurses, occasionally doctors (who sometimes enclosed a publication they had written), students, health educators, social workers, community volunteers, and others, but sometimes they were just sick or troubled people needing support.

I had told my interviewer that the great majority of illnesses are never seen by a doctor; that most primary care is given by one's own family, close friends, and neighbors; that in every community there are key people others turn to for advice, counsel, and support. I explained how I had found ways to identify these natural helpers, lay advisers, health facilitators—I use the terms interchangeably—had offered them courses of basic information in health, and had linked them up with area agencies.

This community health education program began in 1973 in Durham County, its express purpose to teach and strengthen facilitators who would carry on as knowledgeable advisers long after my funding had ended. Conceptually, it evolved directly from my own experiences. In South Africa I had learned that a health service can only become effective in an African culture when professionals understand the basic needs of the people they serve and when they link up with indigenous workers to attend to those needs. In Boston I learned that self-esteem, integral to people's well-being, is fostered by recognizing their strengths rather than their weaknesses and by involving them in their own health care. In both places and in North Carolina I learned that politics, economics, and social class play a very large part in the health of communities, and I learned that it's futile to use short-term grants to raise health status if there's no way to continue the program when funding ends.

I never doubted the presence of caring lay persons in our community, indeed in all communities, or that others would recognize these persons as supportive and would turn to them for advice and counsel. Mark Clay in Bracken Field had convinced me of their presence. But I found Mark by happenstance; I hadn't previously worked out ways to search systematically for natural helpers. We acquired an office in Bragtown to house the program staff—an administrator, a health educator, four community coordinators, and a secretary—and together as a team we planned the details of the program.[2]

The initial method of identifying natural helpers was simple—I added a question to the household survey: "Is there anyone you know around here who is a good person to ask for advice about some health or medical problem—aside from doctors?" This question netted a large number of names. Our field staff asked the same question, taking time for more detailed explanations, at local churches, health and social agencies, community clubs, and other group meetings. They also questioned key persons in the area—teachers, ministers, church mothers, storekeepers, postmasters, beauticians, and field-workers of local service agencies. If the county had not been "dry" at the time, we would have included bartenders. Our coordinators, longtime residents of the same area, knew the people well enough to add extra names. When we had our first group of facilitators, they proved our best source for finding others like themselves. And, finally, we went to the acknowledged leaders of the community and asked them not only to name facilitators, but also to steer us to others as able as themselves to suggest the right people.

Once we had a list of names, we visited these potential facilitators at home and introduced ourselves. We told them their neighbors had identified them as people the community trusted and to whom they went for help and advice. And then we invited them to join a group of natural helpers like themselves and to let us know what additional information would be useful to them so they could help their neighbors even better. We wouldn't be paying them, but we thought they would enjoy meeting each other and having this learning experience.

We gathered many more names than the thirty-nine health facilitators we ended up involving, but we were limited by our budget. Deliberately, we chose to include men and women of a wide range of ages—from sixteen to seventy, most already active in church, club, and other community activities. Two-thirds were women, most often housewives. Of those women who worked a number were in the health field as nurse-aides, family health workers, recreation coordinators, and licensed practical nurses. Three of our men were ministers. Our youngest recruits were still at school; a couple of the oldest were retired. Our most unusual member was widely known as a "root-doctor" (herbalist) about whom I'll say more later. To me it was interesting that some had grandmothers who had been "granny midwives." Our staff was predominantly black and female; it wasn't surprising that the facilitators were too.

When I began to look for financial support to make my ideas a reality, my past experience made me wary of arousing community expectations of long-lasting programs which might well end as soon as the money ran out. To avoid this happening I knew we'd have to train the natural helpers in such a way that they'd continue the work when we were gone, and I had to convince service agencies of my model's potential usefulness so they would pick it up.

Every time I spoke at a meeting, I suggested organizations— health centers, health departments, housing authorities, churches, voluntary agencies—which might find our model beneficial. To keep their interest we used their staff as teachers and resource people in our training, designed videotapes which they could use, set up monthly workshops, and published articles and a guide describing our program.[3] In our last year we wrote a newsletter which we circulated widely. One of the items was a column in which we encouraged readers to send in their queries. It took some time for the seeds to bear fruit, but in the end agencies of all types adopted some aspects of our program.

Our budget allowed us to train only three groups of thirteen facilitators each. Group training went on for three months with about eight evening sessions, and each of these began with light refreshments and a "warm-up"—a game or a song—to put people at ease. Among our many topics were: the role of a health facilitator, the structure and use of the health care system, and common illnesses of children and adults. One part of our teaching emphasized promotion of health and prevention of disease; we called it "Be good to yourself." Here we talked about childhood growth and development, nutrition, smoking, drinking, and sexuality, and we ended with two evenings on first aid.

I was present at every session and led a few—notably the one on smoking. I must have shown how strongly I felt about the harm it causes because another time when we debated about how to change a particular behavior pattern one facilitator said, "Get Dr. Salber on it!" The evening on sexuality was one to remember. Our health educator had arranged for someone she knew to lead the discussion. Informally dressed, he had long hair tied neatly down the back of his neck, and he looked *very* young. Somewhat apprehensively I listened to his forthright language. There were several questions at the end, and I blessed our oldest facilitator, a former schoolteacher, for immediately starting the discussion with a question on homosexuality. But after the session ended, one of the other elderly facilitators approached me to ask shyly, "I didn't want to ask that young man, but would you tell me what a lesbian is?" I wanted the coordinators to get reactions to the lecture and to let me know

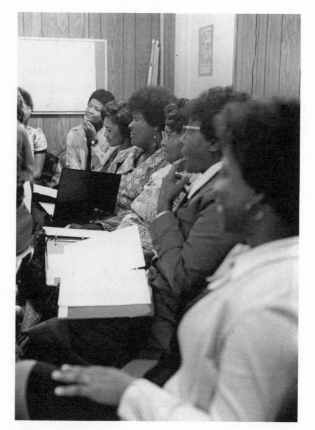

Health facilitator training session

in case we needed to soothe any feelings. Coordinators reported that the older people said *they* "could take it," but they worried about "how the young ones felt." The young ones indicated that it was OK for *them*, but they felt "it might be too much for the older ones."

With the permission of participants, we allowed a few on-lookers at each session, provided they kept silent. Week after week public health nurses, whose home-visiting region coincided with the boundaries of our program area, watched the proceedings. When I asked the reason for their faithfulness, they said it helped them see the people they knew as patients in an entirely new light.

We used staff from my other programs in Community Health Models as we needed them—to give demographic information culled from the health interview survey and to videotape each session so that those who missed a meeting could view it at their convenience. It was a novelty for our participants to be on videotape, and they loved it. (It also strengthened the resolve of our more chubby members to stick to their diets.) We made "trigger tapes" as well as videotapes which we, and later others, used to show what we were trying to accomplish. But important as group sessions were, the fundamental training took place on a one-to-one basis between a coordinator and his or her facilitators.

Before we started to train the facilitators, the coordinators were themselves intensively drilled for their roles. One of their functions was to prepare fact sheets—packets of information on topics asked for by the facilitators or that senior staff thought essential. It was best for coordinators to prepare these sheets and professionals to monitor them since we had to use language easy to understand. Over sixty fact sheets were drawn up on subjects as different as hypertension and housing. Each coordinator, responsible for a certain number of facilitators, met with them at least once a week and developed trusting and enduring relationships.

We also designed a contact sheet for recording the problems residents brought to their facilitators and the suggestions they were given. To evaluate our program we needed the sex, age, and race of each person who consulted a facilitator, but asked for initials rather than names to preserve confidentiality. For me the most moving times came when I read these problems and the solutions offered. A large number of questions were about common illnesses for which the usual advice was to see a doctor. In cases of severe distress or injuries, these lay advisers told residents to go to the hospital emergency room and even drove them there. And, just as a mother will use her judgment with her child, these community mothers (and fathers) at times suggested harmless home remedies or plain aspirin. But we were *not* training lay people to replace physicians; they bore no resemblance to the Chinese "barefoot doctors," nor did they dispense medicines as is common in Third World countries.

Many of the problems were familial, social, and economic, matters unlikely to be brought out in brief visits to a clinic where a prescription can too often replace communication. The age, sex, and occupation of the helpers influenced the type of problem brought to them. For example, our youngest facilitator, a high school football star, was asked for help on teenage sex, difficult schoolwork, lack of recreation facilities, and sports injuries. Our ministers were approached for counsel on marital and family problems as well as on spiritual needs. Middle-aged women were turned to in cases of depression, loneliness, lack of food, marital difficulties, alcoholism, and family care during hospitalization of a mother.

Responses and help proffered were as illuminating as the problems themselves—almost always practical, sympathetic, and true to the shared values of the community. A facilitator once came across a woman and her two small children sitting on the steps of the Department of Social Services, weeping bitterly. The family had come from a far-off town to follow the husband and father to Durham but found he had deserted them. The wife, penniless, appealed to Social Services, who couldn't help her because she wasn't a resident of their county. The woman was desperate. So the soft-hearted facilitator, who had five children of her own, took the family home with her, fed them, comforted them, and sheltered them for several months until she found a job for the mother. I thought then, as I have many other times, that the poor are the most truly generous.

Teenagers were freer in their behavior than the previous generation but still unsure of themselves. One young girl asked of her trusted older adviser, "Should I give in and have sex with my boy friend?" "No," came the answer, "he will lose respect for you." But girls already sexually active were directed to the health department for contraceptive advice and material.

Institutions weren't trusted as much as individuals. One of our facilitators, a clerical worker in the pharmacy department of Duke Hospital, was often consulted by employees who suspected they'd contracted venereal disease. Naively, I enquired why they asked advice of him instead of staff in Duke's employee health service. He told me employees didn't trust the confidentiality of their medical records and avoided reporting symptoms of venereal disease, or emotional disturbances, for fear of losing their jobs.

In times of crisis—when a young daughter suddenly left home, a child became pregnant, a husband was repeatedly unkind to his wife or drank too much, an older person felt overwhelmed by sorrow and loneliness—the helpers gave no specific advice but much comfort. They sat, held hands, and listened. But most often, being activists, they tried to do something practical. If a facilitator didn't know the answer to a question, she went to her coordinator, who in turn could consult with the health educator or the administrator or finally with me. Together we usually produced an answer.

When home remedies were suggested for minor ailments, I checked them, and if I thought they might be harmful—a drop of turpentine on a sugar cube as a cure for worms made me feel uneasy—I sent messages through a coordinator or arranged that the problem be discussed in training. Our root-doctor, a black man of sixty-seven, was known throughout the area but wasn't easy to pin down on any specifics the day I spent more than two hours interviewing him in his home.[4] When he learned that I came from South Africa he warmed up. "Well you come from Africa, and you heard those tales about witch doctors, voodoo, all stuff like that. You'll understand. My daddy's uncle, he was supposed to be a wizard."

In the old days, when there were few doctors or hospitals around, our root-doctor had set fractures, stitched wounds, and treated burns, consumption, and arthritis, but now he seemed

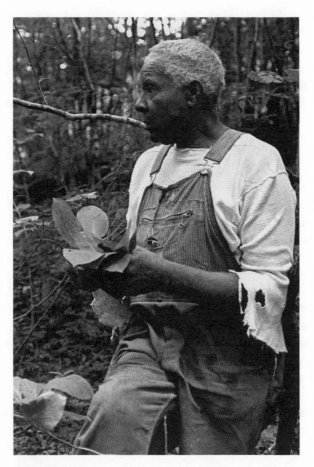

Our root-doctor

to be consulted mostly on money matters, marital disagreements,
interpretation of dreams, and enhancement of sexual potency.
He also admitted to telling fortunes. When I wanted to know
whether he would treat my own arthritis, he smiled and asked
if I had a hundred dollars. He saw no merit in my suggestion
that I should get a professional discount, and I continued to take
aspirin. But he did eventually give us a lesson in herbal lore and

other kinds of folk medicine, some of which I give here with apologies for possible misrepresentation.

Lion's tongue and ratvein were used for rheumatism, heartleaf for heart trouble, berberry root for hives and poison ivy, gall-of-the-earth (nicknamed also boss-of-the-world) for rattlesnake bites, catnip for colds, garlic for worms, and mayapple for constipation. Asthma could be relieved by smoking tansy or by sleeping on a pillow stuffed with rabbit tobacco. For "improving nature" in old men and for young men who were "losing their power," puccoon root—especially if steeped in moonshine—was very effective. But I didn't manage to draw out his treatment for shingles, for which he was famous locally, though he told me a hair-raising tale of a treatment in vogue in his father's time. This involved painting the painful area with the fresh blood of a black chicken ripped open alive or with the blood of a newly severed cat's tail!

Unfortunately for us, Duke's department of public relations responded to the request of a visiting journalist, who was interested in folk medicine, and sent him to us. Nothing would convince him that ours was *not* a program about folk medicine. Nor did he keep his promise that he wouldn't publish anything without my checking it first. He met with some facilitators, including the root-doctor, and for the next several months, as his articles appeared in newspapers in different parts of the country, I got heartrending letters asking for our shingles cure.

The end of each training period was celebrated in a graduation ceremony and awarding of certificates. I remember the first one particularly well since it was held in my home, and Dr. Estes handed out the diplomas. Staff speeches were short but warm, and we were all outshone by one of the facilitators who replied on behalf of the other participants. She talked about the "family night" monthly meetings she and her coordinator had initiated, at which they had a speaker or showed films of an educational nature. All the comments we heard that evening were extremely encouraging:

"After everything has been recorded, do you think we can get this into a book which people can purchase in the future? Because one thing I would like to say is that if a person has the opportunity to get involved in a program like this . . . to try and make the best of it, because we are trying to help yourself and others too."

"The best thing about the program is that it began."

"It has taught me to know that there are people who will help other people who don't have to be welfare people."

"The best thing was that the teaching was done on a grass-roots level where anyone could grasp what was being said."

"The program increased my ability to help other people. It was an open door that I did not know was available." (This from a minister.)

"The worst thing about the program was that it stopped too soon."

To me the best thing was that it *didn't* stop. Others carried on.

Small, modified replicas cropped up in New Zealand, Canada, South Africa, and all over the United States. Some I heard about when their sponsors called or wrote to me asking for materials like our manual, our fact sheets, our published articles, or our consultation and assistance. Others I heard about by chance. At times I learned that a new project didn't know about us but about another program that stemmed from ours. To this day, when I get a call which begins, "You don't know me, but . . ." it's always from someone who wants to know more about the facilitator program.

I once told a group at Bristol University in England that Porirua, New Zealand, had been one of the first places to adapt our model to the needs of its minority populations. A young doctor in the audience challenged me. "I know that program," he said. "I've been there and seen it. The health department is running it." He was surprised to learn that the path to that health department began at our door.

I mention here only a few of the many programs based on our model. A Duke medical student adapted our concept for use among Hmong refugees in Seattle. Other medical students trained Health Helpers as their summer rural health project at a plant manufacturing car mirrors in Bolivar, Tennessee. These students boarded with local residents in Bolivar, and some hosts felt embarrassed in having far less formal education than their boarders. One woman told me she felt uncomfortable having a medical student from New York City in her rural home.

"I bet you know all kinds of things he doesn't," I said to comfort her. She thought a moment and her face lit up. "Well, you know, I couldn't believe he didn't know how long a cow is pregnant!" This was my opportunity to reinforce her rural wisdom in contrast to our urban ignorance. "I don't know either. How long *is* a cow pregnant?" Her answer came with a broad smile. "Why, nine months, of course."

I take special pride in two programs. A black South African friend, who studied public health in Chapel Hill for a year and came to one of our workshops, began identifying and training "child-minders" in Soweto. Many Soweto mothers worked away from home and were forced to leave their infants with hard-pressed neighbors or relatives. Her child-minder program was cited when she joined eighty-three other women who, in 1986, the *Star* newspaper of Johannesburg named South African "Women of the Year."

Closer to home is the program I call the Black Church Project, which is sponsored by the General Baptist State Convention. Our health educator's husband, who sat in on all our group training sessions, directed this church venture which drew its facilitators from church members. Beginning in 1981 three years were spent in educating the community about diseases which hit black people hard, such as hypertension and diabetes, and after that the focus was on preventing illness. Facilitators did their best to persuade their neighbors to stop smoking, to lose weight, to cook with less salt, and to manage stressful situations more efficiently.

The last time I took an active part in their proceedings was about a week after I had broken my right arm. The director had asked me to "inspire" his latest graduates at a banquet honoring them. I told the graduates, truthfully, that I'd have canceled speaking on any other platform than that one.

I don't like books or movies that leave me dangling; I always want to know what happened afterward. So I tell now about the facilitators when our program came to an end. They carried on in their helping roles and kept in touch with those coordinators who remained living in their area. We came together early on at a joyous reunion party, a few years later at the wedding of a coordinator, and last year at a supper. Two of our youngest facilitators had gone on to college; another had some training in a physician associate program. One became a registered nurse, another a hospital administrator, a third a matron in a women's jail. Some took courses in subjects of interest to them—problems of the elderly, nutrition, housing. Many didn't change their previous jobs, but all gained stature in their own and in their community's eyes, and several agencies sought their services. They framed their certificates and displayed them, proudly, on living room walls. A letter I got from a woman prisoner is one example of the effect they had on those they helped.

> I, Sharon, would also like to say that she [the facilitator] is a very good person on the inside as well as on the outside. The other girls and I would like to say that if all the matrons were as understanding as she is, Durham County jail would be very pleasant. She's a hardworking home lady and we admire her. In concluding, we would like to say may she have the best of luck in the near future and we love her.

What was the effect of this program on me? It was an uplifting, satisfying, and joyful project to be in. Uplifting because it proved that one can find compassionate people everywhere that are willing to help others without monetary reward simply because they care; satisfying because the program was successful and continues to be in its many spin-offs; and joyful because how could I be otherwise in the company of so many kindly, capable, good-humored, and loving people. Their philosophy is stated for me in the words of one facilitator who told me, "My husband calls me the community mother."

Don't Send Me Flowers When I'm Dead

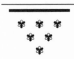

Shortly before I retired from Duke University in mid-1982, I finished writing a book on the lives of forty-five rural, elderly people who were living alone.[1] The men and women I wrote about were residents of Red Hill and Ashton[2]—two adjoining villages occupying about sixty-four square miles in the Piedmont section of North Carolina, and many had spent their entire lives in the area. Each village had a few modest stores, gas stations, lunch counters, a post office, several unpretentious churches, small farms, tobacco barns—some still made of logs—and with few exceptions rather plain, single-family houses. A sizable number of families, particularly black families, had no car, telephone, indoor running water or indoor toilet.

The book's title came from one of the women I interviewed, who said to me, "I tell people, 'Don't send me flowers when I'm dead. I want them now. It wouldn't do me two cents worth of good after I'm dead to put me in my grave and put a pile of flowers on me as big as this house. If you've got a flower you want me to have, give it to me while I'm living.'"

The idea of writing this book evolved slowly. As with my earlier book, "Caring and Curing: Community Participation in Health Services,"[3] it was triggered by the scientific research I had been doing. During analysis of our household interview survey, I had become aware that rural elderly were what professional jargon calls a high-risk group. In simpler terms they were a part of the sicker, poorer, and more neglected sections of our society. I believed that among the elderly those who lived alone would be the most vulnerable, and I wanted to see what community services were needed to help people remain in their own

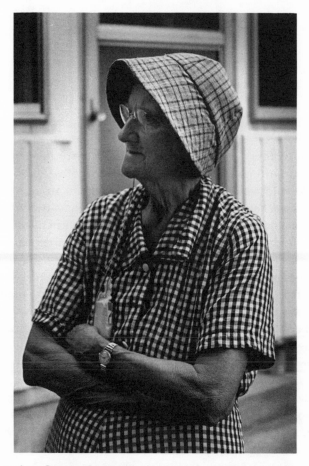

Don't send me flowers when I'm dead. I want them now

homes if that was their wish. However, once I began to know these elderly people, my purpose broadened. As I realized how much they had to teach me and others, I searched for a way to pass on the lessons of their lives to a wider audience than readers of medical journals. The situation matched my uncertainty on how best to write about the Bracken Field Housing Project residents, and once again I chose to capture voices through the use of unstructured tape-recorded interviews.

I hadn't realized in 1975, when I began my interviews, how involved I would become, but for the next five years I made at least one annual visit to each of the people I interviewed. On the first introductory visit, I was armed with a tape recorder and accompanied by Becky, a dedicated assistant who, fortunately, knew the area intimately. At that time the people we met couldn't believe that their lives could possibly be of interest to us, but when they were convinced that I wanted nothing better than to listen to them, they responded readily. When I showed how important they were to me by bringing two skilled photographer friends to them to record their faces, their homes, and their landscape, they were delighted.[4] Our attention gratified their need to be remembered and bolstered their self-esteem, their pride in the hard work they had done, the way in which they had managed their lives, their dignified acceptance that God had chosen them for a long life.

Before I met the people I was to interview, I expected to find them socially isolated, lonely, and despondent, but I was mistaken. I hadn't realized that these people in their 70s and 80s had known each other from their first grade at school and attended the same church services. Their lives revolved around their families, their land, their work, and their church. But to me their most striking characteristic was their independence.

As a doctor I was used to giving advice—at times unsought—and found that I was wrong once again in assuming that logic was more powerful than sentiment and personality. When I discovered that Rose Chambers, aged eighty-two, was twin sister to George Ross, I asked her why she and her brother didn't move in together. She told me, gently, that they'd discussed the matter several times, but each wanted the other to do the moving. Mr. Ross confided to me later that he didn't want to report on his movements to his sister, and Mrs. Chambers couldn't bear to leave the house she had lived in from the day of her marriage.

Once I was asked if I would take six University of North Carolina medical students to some of the homes I visited. My first choice was Mrs. Woods, then in her early 80s. I chose Sally

Woods because she was crippled with arthritis—her back was crooked and the joints of her hands and legs obviously affected. The students agreed that if they'd seen her only in a clinic setting, they would have recommended institutional living, believing she could not possibly live by herself. But in her own surroundings they marveled at her spotless house, although she walked around holding onto the furniture. She told them she did not like to use her walker because she didn't want to become too dependent on it. The students, impressed by her spunk, but awkward in their questions, confined what they asked to her medical condition. As Mrs. Woods and I chatted warmly about her week's activities, they gradually relaxed and genuinely appreciated her display of forty pots of healthy African violets and the needlework she was still doing. I told them that if Mrs. Woods fell she knew she would have to lie there until someone came by to pick her up and that a neighbor checked on her each noon and her son each evening at six. She was willing to trade the risk of falling for continued independence. On the way home the students began to talk to me about their own grandparents.

As fiercely independent as Mrs. Woods was Anne Parker. Also in her eighties, Mrs. Parker now depended on a neighbor to plant her vegetables, but she continued to pick them herself by sitting on a chair light enough to move between the rows. Her supply of preserves was as much a matter of pride of management and a means of exchange as it was a source of food. Rarely would a clinic visit bring out such facts—as important as a routine medical history and examination. She liked to feed anyone who seemed hungry and as a result had the problem of twenty-eight wild cats living in her garden. We arranged to have the cats removed.

I had known that successful, independent living was closely tied to adequate housing, including indoor plumbing, which in turn was related to income level. In our household survey we had used the absence of certain amenities of living as proxy measures for poverty: a family car, a telephone, indoor running water, and an indoor toilet.[5] It was in these interviews that the true value of appliances, conveniences, and particularly indoor plumbing, to older, rural people became painfully clear. They were stoic and uncomplaining, but it was hard to collect water from a spring or a neighbor's well, to go outdoors in very cold weather to use a toilet, to live in poorly maintained, inadequately insulated houses, to wash clothes by hand or in an antiquated washing machine, to lack a telephone, to choose between keeping warm in winter or skimping on food, and all these deficiencies hastened institutionalization when their frailty increased.

These stalwart people brushed aside deprivations by telling me they were "old-timey" and used to living the hard way. All the same when Lola Buchanan, who lived in a tumbledown frame shack, was given a new house by the children of a woman she had devotedly nursed for many years, her delight in turning on her kitchen faucet to wash her dishes moved me to tears.

Walter Jordan, a black man of seventy-one, was also matter-of-fact about his house. He lived in a two-room, ramshackle log cabin, his few clothes hanging from nails in the wall. His brother, a chauffeur in Connecticut, had given him a car, a telephone, installed electricity (the wires were exposed and a single naked light bulb hung crookedly from the ceiling), and sent him a radio and a television set. But the cabin, which he rented for fifteen dollars a month, had no water supply nor toilet of any kind. He used the facilities of his landlady or the woods around him. I had great difficulty understanding Mr. Jordan because he was chewing a big wad of tobacco throughout the interview, and he had taken out his dentures to avoid staining them with tobacco juice.

On one of my follow-up interviews I found that Mr. Jordan had moved to another county, and I followed him there. Living in a newly furnished trailer owned by his brother, Mr. Jordan's appearance was as transformed as his dwelling place. He was wearing his dentures, and I suddenly saw a handsome man, his dignity, previously hidden to me, now revealed by his new clothes and surroundings.

I used to tell students that too many cups of early morning coffee could be a hazard in fieldwork. But despite taking my

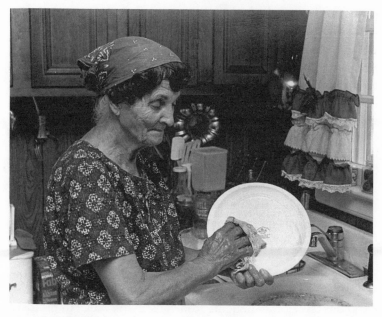

The joy of running water

own advice, I often had to ask permission to use a bathroom; I knew the location of each one with a flush toilet. (I had heard too many tales of black widow spiders in outhouses to try those.) I asked Mr. Jordan if I could use his bathroom and he replied, "Which one?"

One of my regular questions was about food stamps. I found that many people who are eligible for food stamps don't get them. Some people, too proud to apply, despised the welfare system, thought most welfare recipients were undeserving, and that welfare had ruined the nation. On the other hand some didn't apply for food stamps because they felt others needed them more. And several didn't apply because they could hardly read and avoided forms they didn't understand.

I knew of course that blacks and whites formed their own distinct communities, but I hadn't realized fully the extent of this separateness or that all the churches were segregated. It was strange to me to see a black Baptist church on one side of the road facing a white Baptist church on the opposite side. Toward the end of my study period a senior center opened in the fellowship hall of a white church. Although this was an integrated meeting place, even here I noticed that blacks sat together in one group, whites in another. I went to a few black services and to two white ones. I remember well one of the white services. I had read that Southern white religion focused on personal sin and salvation and deliberately disengaged itself from secular affairs, in contrast to European Protestant churches which concerned themselves also with social responsibility.[6] Sure enough the Baptist minister's rhetoric was powerful and preoccupied with the personal salvation of individual members of his flock who had sinned. But the black pastors attended to secular as well as spiritual affairs, urging their parishioners to vote in political elections.

The relationships between some black and white elderly women seemed warm, perhaps because most of the black women had brought up not only their own families, but also the children of white families, and had helped older, sick, white folk. On the other hand contacts between black men and white families were seldom intimate. And as hard as life was for whites, it was harder yet for blacks.

Bill Parrish, aged sixty-eight, described his life to me. When he was in the second grade, his mother took him out of school and put him to work for a farmer for twenty cents a day. He would plow, starting when the sun rose. Barely nine years old, he walked a mile and a half to work on Monday morning and stayed all week. His father had deserted the family leaving his mother to keep them going through her "day work." Mr. Parrish was very pleased when he finally retired and did only a few odd jobs, cutting grass for the white folks or clearing a walkway in the snow. "When I ain't working," he told me, "sometimes I go down to the boathouse and listen to the white folks talk. I don't make talk when they talk; I be quiet. When they say something embarrass, something wrong that I think I know better

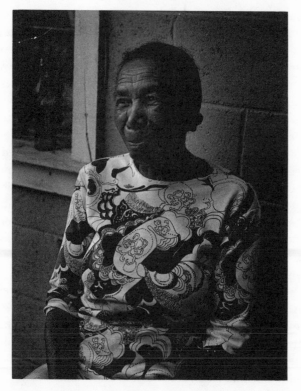

Nobody such as me didn't own no land worth nothing

than that, I don't say nothing. I don't meddle in they talk." (I was reminded of a conversation with some black, South African friends. The boss remained unaware of softly mouthed maledictions, they said, as long as each sentence ended with the obligatory, loud "Baas" [Master] or "Madam.")

Ola Hill also described old and more recent times. "My parents farmed, 'bacco, corn, 'tatoes, and stuff like that. Yes ma'am on the white people's land. See, 'long then nobody such as me didn't own no land worth nothing 'cause we wasn't able. Our mothers had to wash and iron and clean up and cook and all such as that for the white people." At seventy-two she still does day work for a family whose children she helped to rear and told me how good they were to her. Again South Africa comes to mind for I knew many families there, including my own, who maintained the same unequal but warm interdependency. I know of more than one South African family who, having emigrated, sent air tickets to former maids so they could attend the weddings of the children to whom they had been second mothers.

While I'd been mistaken in thinking that these rural men and women would be socially isolated, I also hadn't recognized fully the special kind of grievous loneliness that death of a spouse brought to their elderly survivors. Later, I realized that dirt farming more than most occupations brought husbands and wives constantly together, working side by side until one partner died, leaving the other only half a person. Nor had I known that the loss of a mate was especially hard on the men. They told me how good their marriages had been, how much their wives had helped them, how awful lonesome it now was. It was not that women didn't feel their loss as keenly, but they managed better. They kept busy with daily household duties, looking after their flowers, putting up preserves, going to quilting bees, helping with grandchildren. By that time most men had slowed down on their usual outdoor work activities.

Most of the bereaved men didn't want to marry again, but one man, white, sixty-seven-year-old Will Clark, desperately wanted another wife. Shortly after my first visit to him, he answered my Christmas card. "Dear Friend, will answer your sweet letter with best wishes and a Happy New Year. . . . I want to ask you a favor. If you know some nice widow that would like to marry me and share my nice home and flowers and housekeep, I would love for you to let me know. Any age from forty to sixty-five years old would be great."

I did my very best, exploring senior centers (which always have a preponderance of women), but failed to find him a wife. Fortunately, he found one himself and was very happy. I happened to visit three weeks later and recognized immediately from the look of pleasure on his face, and from his new dentures, what had transpired. His bride was away deciding which personal possessions from her old home she should bring back with her, but Mr. Clark showed me her photograph and smilingly confided: "She done me more good than every doctor that I've ever seen for years, and it done me more good than all the medicines ever I took. I feel just as good as I felt when I was fifty years old."

Often I wished that doctors and social workers would assess patients and clients in the home setting, and I wished that their visits would be longer, more explanatory, more understanding. Ella Daniels, who was blind, related a poignant story of a new reading machine her case worker had sent her. In contrast to the early machine she had had many years previously, the new one was too complicated for her to operate, and she had to send it back.

When eighty-three-year-old, white George Ross went to a hospital to have his operation, he was puzzled that two doctors besides his surgeon examined him. He was too shy to ask why, and no one thought to explain. Mr. Ross had no bank account and brought all the cash he owned in a pocket of his trousers when he returned for his postoperative checkup. He paid the $900 bill, was told he'd get a refund from Medicare, and received $665. To his great surprise, he then got bills from each of the two additional doctors who'd examined him. He paid those bills also but was bewildered and resentful about the extra doctors and never returned to the hospital. He shared his suspicions with me: "If you got me doing a job of work for you and I come in there and do it and then drag in somebody else and stick their name on it, now what is that? Now it runs in my mind them doctors that come in there, they may be what you'd call junky people somewhere; they got no job, probably cain't get nary one, and he likes 'em and he'll take 'em in. A poor man like I am cain't go to the hospital and come back home and live. It took all the money I had to pay the doctors."

Over and over again I heard these independent people express their dread of nursing homes. This gnawing worry I understood

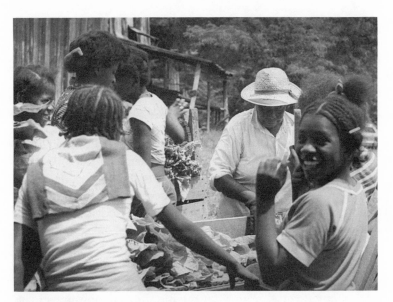

Grandmother and granddaughters preparing tobacco for curing

well, for it is the overwhelming fear of all of us who are getting older and cannot be sure of what awaits us.

I didn't interview people who were in nursing homes, but I did speak to a few in rest homes. The owners were kindly people, but the residents didn't do much smiling or talking. Mostly they just sat quietly. One of the rest-home owners expressed the situation succinctly. "They really do nothing all day." The contrast between them and the independent residents of Red Hill/ Ashton was immense. While these free-living men and women remained active and could put the thoughts of future incapacity out of their minds, life was still sweet to them.

Country people have a great sense of fun and enjoy a hearty laugh. Since we have eight grandchildren ourselves, I can't resist sharing this illustrative quotation. "I ain't got but one child, but High Lord, I got one child and he got fourteen children and then he got twenty-one grandchildren, and you know I got a happy life to live. I look at my son sometimes and I say, 'Lord ha' mercy. If I had two or three children and they had as many children as you got, I would've been head over heels with children wouldn't I?' I'm happy just like I am."

Each time I saw my friends, over the years of my visiting before the book was done, I added a few more words to the interviews. These people, with their openness, their integrity, their kindness, their unpretentiousness, their absence of greed, had become close to my heart. I began to feel that even writing a book was not enough to change the attitudes of the young people, the professionals, and the legislators I wanted to influence. I needed to engage myself on a more personal level—to use my voice to relay the voices of those I heard, as often and whenever the opportunity arose. So, after the book was published, I began to give a series of readings from the book and invited discussions with many diverse groups. Of the hundreds of questions I was asked, five remain uppermost in my mind.

The first was that of a health education student, and it shocked me. I was talking of Will Clark, his great need of a wife, the vain efforts I had made to help him, when she put up her hand. "Why did you go to so much trouble for him?" she asked. Indignant as I was at her lack of sensitivity, I couldn't help but give a lecture, and with some heat reminded her that our careers depend on the cooperation of the people we work with. Without their help we wouldn't get our degrees, earn our fees, write our articles, publish our books. I asked her, "How would *you* feel if there was a knock on *your* door and some stranger said to you, 'Hello. I'm from X university and I'm doing a survey on health habits. I want to ask you a few questions, but I won't keep you long.' "

The second question came from a white, middle-class, sophisticated urban woman. She asked whether I had repeated my study with better-off, city people and suggested that being elderly and alone might be harder for them than for simpler, more contented, rural people. I told her I had not interviewed

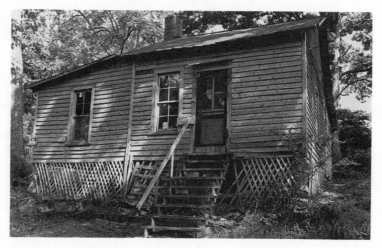

*If you're old, and sick, and alone, it's better
to be rich than poor*

well-to-do, urban elderly, but from my experience with poor,
rural survivors I could honestly say, "If you're old, and sick,
and alone, it's better to be rich than poor."

The third question I remember because it floored me. I didn't
know the answer. A young minister wanted to know, "How did
you discover the richness in these people's lives?" I have thought
of that question many times and am still no nearer a better
answer than I gave at the time. "I listened."

The fourth question showed typical audience disbelief. "Were
those rural people really as content with their lot as you make
them out to be?" At one reading, when I was asked this question,
it was answered for me by a young woman who got up to speak
holding an open copy of my book in her hand. She identified
herself as the granddaughter of Bill Hall (by then almost ninety),
told the group that what I said was true, and asked me to read
the section on her grandfather.

The fifth question came frequently though not as often as I
asked it of myself. "Were these people's lives improved in any
way because you interviewed them?" Yes, Becky and I helped

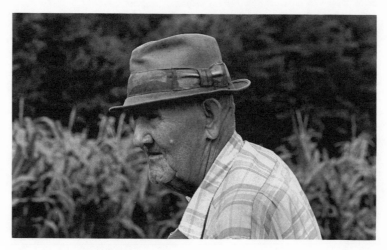

Bill Hall still planting corn

a number of individuals. We got them onto food stamps and Supplemental Security Income (SSI). We delivered needed medication to patients who had no transportation. We persuaded an agency to repair the rickety steps and broken porch of our blind friend. We took a beloved pet to the vet for treatment and in another home removed troublesome cats. We bought hand-made quilts for more money than they could fetch at church bazaars. But these were specific and limited attempts at helping and could have been done by anybody. Our other actions are harder to assess but perhaps in the long run more important. It's difficult to put a value on friendship, on affection, on caring, but the people I knew seemed to appreciate the many hours I spent with them, my continuing visits and Christmas letters, my obvious interest in their welfare, and my attempts to soften the system for their benefit. When some of those I interviewed died, I got letters from their children telling me so and report-ing that they and their parents were happy that I had not for-gotten them when the study ended. Like the people of Bracken Field, it meant a lot to them to be in a book and have their words quoted.

I try particularly to do readings for health professionals (and have done many of these) and for legislators (only one so far). The readings provide an easy way to point out deficiencies in our system which can be remedied. I tell doctors of a call I got one day from a young resident in Duke's Family Medicine Program. He had become Mrs. Daniels's doctor. She told him he was only the second doctor who had ever come to visit her at home. I was the first, she said, and pointed to my Christmas card (which she couldn't see) on her mantelpiece. I speak about the inadequacies of our fee-for-service system, of the inequality between health services for the rich and the poor, about the niggardly provisions of social welfare programs, about the fear of nursing homes and the great need for home-based care. And over and over again I stress the tremendous importance of the social security system. However badly off some of these rural elderly are, their parents had been worse off without social security.

I bought enough copies of the published book to give a copy to each person I interviewed and to all those who had helped me in my task. I was delighted at the pleasure these elderly residents of Redhill/Ashton showed in seeing and receiving their own personal copies of the book, in looking at the photographs, and in hearing me read their words back to them.

But at the same time I had some personal sadness. I needed to deal with the letdown feeling that I always get when an intense involvement with a community over a long period has ended. I needed the lift of laughter. Musing, I recalled my last few conversations with Betty Hunt, one of the women I had interviewed. Chuckling at the memory, I wrote myself a story on some of the exchanges between the two of us, and I called it "Design Dresses and Rabbit Droppings."

For a long time I owned a dress fashioned by Hannae Mori—a well-known Japanese dress designer. The dress was an indulgence. I had been going to meetings of the American Cancer

Society, held in the Waldorf Astoria Hotel in New York City for many years. Every time I looked at the Hannae Mori shop in the hotel lobby. Her beautiful silk dresses were too expensive for me, but the polyester dresses on sale were very tempting, and I succumbed. The fabric of the dress I bought, with its pattern of diagonal stripes in navy and two shades of rose, was unusual, but the simplicity of the shirtwaist style made it suitable to wear both for meetings and work.

This was the dress I was wearing one day when I visited Mrs. Hunt. I had marveled many times that poor as so many of these rural people were no one asked for any favors. Always direct in her speech, however, Betty Hunt startled me with her remark: "I would take that dress right off your back if I could!" "No need," I replied, "I'll bring it to you next time I visit." Mrs. Hunt addressed herself to my assistant. "That's what she says but she doesn't mean it." Though reassured that if I said it I meant it, she remained unconvinced.

For a brief moment I toyed with the idea of driving home (forty some miles) in my underwear and even imagined the conversation I might have with a traffic cop but decided the idea was impractical. Lingering a while and chatting, I took a closer look at Mrs. Hunt's homemade, shirtwaist dress of faded printed cotton, cut loosely and showing signs of many wearings. Though my dress might be a little snug over her bosom and upper arms, I thought it would fit.

A week or so later I washed the dress, said goodbye to it with a tinge of regret and gave it to Mrs. Hunt. Her face lit up with pleasure while we examined her admiringly from all angles. She told us then that she had not been able to attend her church homecoming, "for people dressed up so," and she had nothing suitable to wear. It was my turn to ask a favor. "Can I have a photograph of you in this dress to remember you by?"

So many times I had come home after interviewing the old people for my book, feeling ashamed and guilty because I had so much and they had so little. This time I felt good. Two weeks later Mrs. Hunt sent me a color snapshot, taken by her niece.

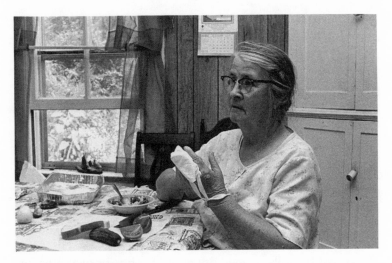

Telling the folk medicine story

She was smiling and happy, in sharp contrast to another photo-graph I have of her with down-turned mouth.

The last time I saw Mrs. Hunt was when I brought her an inscribed copy of my book. While glad to see the book, she asked, hesitantly, "How much is it?" and was relieved to learn it was a gift. (Every person I interviewed and to whom I gave a copy reacted the same way.) Because I had changed all their names in the book, I showed her what her "book name" was, which pages were about her, and read aloud a part of what she'd told me. And then I chided her gently for not allowing me to share with my readers the story of Mrs. Brown. "You shouldn't have listened to me," she said. "You should have put it in." "But you told me to turn that thing [the tape recorder] off." "You should have told it anyhow."

The story she had told me was about folk medicine in the area, a story of an elderly lady of her acquaintance. This lady, whom I called Mrs. Brown, had suffered from arthritis for many years; from time to time she went to her doctor for pills to relieve her discomfort. Once when her grandson of seven or eight was spending the summer with her, she used him to run her errands.

Waking up one morning and feeling her joints to be stiffer and more painful than usual, she sent the child to the doctor for a refill of her medication. It was a good two-mile walk, and Johnny was reluctant. Mrs. Brown insisted, and Johnny took the empty pill box. However, unknown to his grandmother, before he left the house the little boy sneaked into the kitchen and put some flour into a rolled up scrap of newspaper.

Agreeing to be back quickly, Johnny strolled through the woods to a neighboring farm where he had often seen rabbits. Finding what he sought, he rolled the round dung pellets in flour, filled his box, and sauntered about for the period he reckoned it would take to walk to and from the doctor's office. His grandmother rewarded him with two of his favorite cookies and began her treatment. She remarked later to Mrs. Hunt and others that the pills seemed different in consistency and flavor; furthermore she found them far more effective than usual. A staunch churchgoer, who had unwillingly stayed away from church on account of her infirmities, Mrs. Brown returned as soon as possible—taking Johnny with her. By chance she spotted her doctor walking past her pew. Thanking him effusively, she told him how much better she felt since he had changed her medicine; soon she would be asking for more. After five minutes of conversation with her doctor, Mrs. Brown realized that Johnny had been her pharmacist! What had he given her? A spanking with a switch from a dogwood tree brought out a pained confession.

We both laughed, relishing the anecdote. "After all," mused Mrs. Hunt, "rabbits eat grass and fresh vegetables, healthy things. Perhaps that medicine really was better than the one from the doctor. I don't know if it's true, but I heard that she used it again!"

Afterword

He who learns from children—what is he like?
One who eats sour grapes and drinks fresh wine.
And he who learns from an old man—what is he like?
He who eats ripe grapes and drinks vintage wine.
—Sayings of the Fathers

Looking back from what Ronald Blythe calls the view in winter, I know that my early participation in the South African health center movement made me an enthusiastic proponent of social medicine and a doctor to underprivileged communities. In America I continued on that path.

At medical school I was taught the importance of biology in the causation of illness. In Umtata and in Durban I learned that politics, economics, culture, and tradition are just as important. In Boston and in North Carolina I discovered that self-esteem is directly related to wellness. And, in every job I did, I saw that medicine by itself can't control sickness due to poverty, bad housing, lack of education, environmental hazards, and racial and class discrimination.

Samuel Johnson once wrote: "We are all prompted by the same motives, all deceived by the same fallacies, all animated by hope, obstructed by danger, entangled by desire, and seduced by pleasure." We doctors are a product of our society, true enough, but we also belong to a compassionate profession which should be able to guard us from commercialization and help us to retain our humanity. It is disgraceful that the least care so often goes to those who need it most, but who cannot pay their bills. And it is shameful that still today South Africa and America are linked together as the only two industrialized

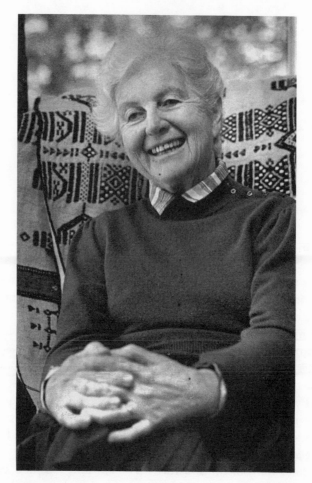

Looking back from the view in winter

countries of the world that do not have a national health program in place.

We older people want to review our lives and tell our stories to our grandchildren, and even to strangers when we think we have something to teach them—hence this book. As the pattern of people and events falls into place over the years, we gain perspective and understanding. My own review shamed me into

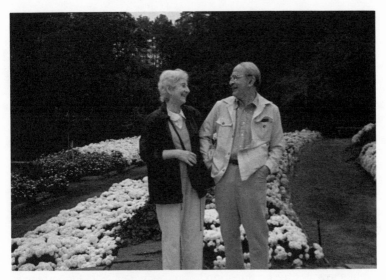

*The struggles have been strengthening
and the rewards immense*

seeing how long-standing and petty many of my resentments
had been, and I was relieved that bringing these vexations into
the open wiped them out. It has been an intense, uplifting emotional experience to relive my life as a young woman, a wife, a
mother (though the children crossed out most of what I put in
about them), and a doctor. I believe that being a mother made
me a gentler, more sympathetic doctor and that being a doctor
made me a more loving and understanding mother. It isn't easy
for women to combine motherhood and work outside the home,
and we often feel guilty, but reviewing enabled me to acknowledge that my well-being depended not only on the love of my
family but also on the satisfaction I got in being useful to some
of society's disregarded people. Most of all I recognized what a
privileged life I had led in being able to earn my living, and
express my values, in doing the work I wanted to do. I have
never had a job in which I wasn't completely involved or that
didn't enlarge my understanding or that failed to cement my

connectedness with other human beings. Can one ask for more than this?

Now seventy-two, I rejoice that our family includes eight grandchildren and that retirement has not meant a loss of interest in former colleagues, students, and programs. My health facilitator model still flourishes; at times I'm asked to help and to tell of its beginnings. As I age along with them, I follow the declining years of the rural elderly in North Carolina I've got to know so well, and I continue to do my "readings" about them. Young students still come to tap my store of memories, and some community connections, though now more distant, remain. As one of 200 guests, I went to the twentieth anniversary of the Bracken Field Health Center in Boston and joyfully witnessed the splendid growth of the people who taught me so much. As I listened to their speeches, I recalled the ancient rabbi's answer to the question, "Who is wise?": "He who learns from every man." I wondered if I had emphasized this message sufficiently to my students or that other teaching that wisdom without action was not enough: "He whose deeds exceed his wisdom, his wisdom shall endure."

Thinking of my youthful days, I see that the goals of the young woman I once was (and still am inside) stay essentially unaltered. If I could live my life over again, I would change little in my past, for the struggles have been strengthening and the rewards immense. In my own small domain I have done what I could, and in my personal life I am content.

Only South Africa remains a tragic wound, though we emigrated over thirty years ago and 8000 miles separates us. The words of Peter Sacks, a South African poet, stir me deeply.

> You take your sorrow with you when you leave.
> However wide the sea or sky between,
> the journey's end will bring you no reprieve.

As with him, I took my sorrow with me when we left.

Notes

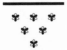

Preface

1. J. W. Cell, *The Highest Stage of White Supremacy: The Origins of Segregation in South Africa and the American South* (New York: Cambridge University Press, 1982), p. ix.
2. E. J. Salber, *Caring and Curing: Community Participation in Health Services* (New York: Neale Watson Academic Publications, 1975).
3. E. J. Salber, *Don't Send Me Flowers When I'm Dead: Voices of Rural Elderly* (Durham, N.C.: Duke University Press, 1983).
4. *Two Dogs and Freedom: Children of the Townships Speak Out* (Braamfontein: Ravan Press and the Open School, 1986), pp. 54–55.
5. R. Blythe, *The View in Winter: Reflections on Old Age* (New York: Harcourt Brace Jovanovich, 1979), p. 29.
6. R. P. Warren, *Brother to Dragons: A Tale in Verse and Voices* (New York: Random House, 1979), p. 130.

Becoming a Doctor

1. R. E. Kirsch, ed., *The Forman Years.* (Cape Town: Department of Medicine UCT, 1984).
2. R. M. Morantz, C. S. Pomerlau, and C. H. Fenichel, eds., *In Her Own Words: Oral History of Women Physicians* (New Haven and London: Yale University Press, 1982), pp. 45–119.
3. L. Thomas, *The Youngest Science: Notes of a Medicine-Watcher* (New York: Viking Press, 1983), pp. 26–35.
4. By 1986 the staff, services, and facilities were almost completely integrated and used for all patients—75 percent of whom were black. S. R. Benatar, "Medicine and Health Care in South Africa," *The New England Journal of Medicine* 315 (1986): 527–532.

Sakkie and the Family

1. E. Roux, *Time Longer Than Rope: A History of the Black Man's Struggle for Freedom in South Africa* (London: Victor Gollanz, 1948), pp. 25–31.

2. E. Roux, pp. 61–85.
3. D. Denoon with B. Nyeko and the advice of J. B. Webster, *Southern Africa since 1800* (New York: Praeger Publishers, 1973), pp. 177–178.
4. G. M. Fredrickson, *White Supremacy: A Comparative Study in American & South African History* (New York: Oxford University Press, 1981), pp. 255–257.
5. H. T. Phillips, *An Inter-Racial Study of Trends in Public Health in the City of Cape Town* (M.D. thesis, University of Cape Town, 1955).
6. M. Horrell, ed., *Survey of Race Relations in South Africa 1981* (Johannesburg: South African Institute of Race Relations 1982), p. 227.
7. C. Cooper, S. Motala, et al., *Survey of Race Relations in South Africa 1983* (Johannesburg: South African Institute of Race Relations 1984), p. 242.

Port Elizabeth: My First Job

1. While writing the final draft of my manuscript, I came across two extraordinary books on the early history of South Africa. Sarah Gertrude Millin's book alerted me to Anthony Trollope's account of his travels through South Africa in 1877. S. G. Millin, *The South Africans* (New York: Boni & Liveright, 1927); A. Trollope, *South Africa*, vols. 1 and 2 (London: Dawsons of Pall Mall, reprinted 1968).
2. Athol Fugard, the well-known South African playwright who still lives in Port Elizabeth, has vividly described the lives of poor blacks, coloreds, and whites in his plays. Korsten is the background for his play "The Blood Knot" which appears in a collection of his plays: A. Fugard, "The Blood Knot," in *Boesman and Lena: And Other Plays* (Cape Town, Oxford University Press, 1980), pp. 3–97.
3. The money I sent home, plus my professional fees earned as court witness (including the per diem allowance for board and lodging which I didn't have to pay) covered the debt. My father insisted on returning the money to me before I left South Africa to join Harry.

Umtata: Rural Poverty

1. Cattle given to the family of the bride bind the marriage contract and give the right of ownership of children of the marriage to the husband. Cattle were a man's wealth and his most treasured possession.
2. W. H. Hutt, "The Economic Position of the Bantu in South Africa," in I. Shapera, ed., *Western Civilization and the Natives of South Africa: Studies in Culture Contact* (London: George Routledge and Sons, 1934), pp. 195–237.
3. M. Susser and V. P. Cherry, "Health and Health Care Under Apartheid," *Journal of Public Health Policy* 3 (1982): 455–475.
4. T. More, translated into English by R. Robynson in 1551, *Utopia* (New York: Heritage Press, 1935), p. 155.

Cape Town: 1941

1. The United States has only recently instituted ambulatory surgery (to save expensive in-patient care); Third World countries with poorer populations and fewer resources have long taken this method for granted.

Durban: Health Center Practice

1. Union of South Africa. Report of the National Health Services Commission on the Provision of an Organized National Health Service for all sections of the People of the Union of South Africa 1942–1944, Union of South Africa Government Printer, Pretoria, 1944.
2. S. L. Kark and G. W. Steuart, eds., *A Practice of Social Medicine: A South African Team's experiences in Different African Communities* (Edinburgh and London, E. and S. Livingstone, 1962).
3. E. J. Salber and E. S. Bradshaw, "Birth Weights of South African Babies," *British Journal of Social Medicine* 5 (1951): 113–119.
4. J. Cassel, "A Comprehensive Health Program Among South African Zulus," in *Health, Culture and Community: Case Studies of Public Reactions to Health Programs,* ed. B. D. Paul and W. B. Miller (New York: Russell Sage Foundation, 1955), pp. 15–41.
5. B. Gampel, "The Hilltops' Community," in S. L. Kark and G. W. Steuart, eds., *A Practice of Social Medicine* (Edinburgh and London, E. and S. Livingstone, 1962), pp. 292–308.
6. For an extensive bibliographic essay on South Africa see Robert Coles' notes to his chapter on "Race and Nationalism: South Africa," in his book *The Political Life of Children* (Boston and New York: Atlantic Monthly Press, 1986), pp. 319–326. See also J. Lelyveld, *Move Your Shadow: South Africa, Black and White* (New York: Times Books, Random House, 1985); and A. Benjamin, ed., *Winnie Mandela: Part of My Soul Went with Him* (New York: W. W. Norton, 1985).
7. C. W. De Kiewiet, *A History of South Africa: Social & Economic* (London: Oxford University Press, 1941), pp. 208–245.
8. *Umeqo*: a psychologic illness or an explanation of chronic ulcers on limbs or of arthritis attributed to contact with poisoned earth or objects placed by an ill-wisher.
9. *Inyoni*: literally a bird, is the African term for severe childhood gastroenteritis, supposedly caused by a pregnant woman walking over a piece of ground on which some ill-wisher has thrown bad medicine which includes part of the "bird of lightning."
10. H. T. Phillips and H. D. Cohn, "The Domiciliary Care of Sick Persons as Part of a Comprehensive Health and Medical Care Programme," *South African Medical Journal* 28 (1954): 613–616.

11. G. W. Gale, "The Aftermath: The 'Gluckman' Report—An Abiding Value" in H. Gluckman, *Abiding Values: Speeches and Addresses* (Johannesburg: Caxton, 1970), pp. 495–518.
12. H. J. Giger, "The Meaning of Community Oriented Primary Care in the American Context," in E. Connor and F. Mullan, eds., *Community Oriented Primary Care: New Directions for Health Services Delivery* (Washington, D.C.: Institute of Medicine Conference Proceedings, National Academy Press, 1983), pp. 60–90.

Cape Town: 1954

1. C. W. De Kiewiet, *The Anatomy of South African Misery* (London: Oxford University Press, 1956), p. 1.
2. H. T. Phillips, *An Inter-racial Study of Trends in Public Health in the City of Cape Town.* (M.D. thesis, University of Cape Town, 1956).
3. The American M.D.—the U.S. qualifying degree—is not the same as the South African M.D. which is an academic, postgraduate degree. However, my U.S. colleagues invariably believe I graduated in 1955, the year I got my M.D., and not in 1938, the year I got my qualifying M.B., Ch. B.
4. E. J. Salber, *Studies in South African Infant Growth: Illustrated by Comparative Analyses of Groups of European, Coloured, Bantu and Indian Babies from Birth to One Year.* (M.D. Thesis, University of Cape Town, 1955).
5. S. L. Kark and J. Chesler, "A Comparative Study of Infant Mortality in Five Communities," in S. L. Kark and G. W. Steuart, eds., *A Practice of Social Medicine* (Edinburgh and London: E. and S. Livingstone, 1962), pp. 114–134.

Emigrating

1. Ronald Blythe acquaints us with the extreme example of the poet Clare who couldn't function when shifted three miles from his native landscape. R. Blythe, *Characters and Their Landscapes* (New York: Harcourt Brace Jovanovich, 1982), p. 1.
2. For a vivid and moving account of Jewish life in Czarist Russia, and of the frantic exodus and resettlement of these Jews, particularly in the United States, see A. Manners, *Poor Cousins* (Greenwich, Conn: Fawcett Publications, 1973).

Settling Down at Harvard

1. E. J. Salber, P. G. Stitt, and J. G. Babbott, "Patterns of Breast Feeding: 1. Factors Affecting the Frequency of Breast Feeding in the Newborn Period," *The New England Journal of Medicine* 259 (1958): 707–713; Salber et al., "Patterns

of Breast Feeding: 2. Duration of Feeding and Reasons for Weaning," *The New England Journal of Medicine* 260 (1959): 310–315.

2. E. J. Salber, E. Goldman, M. Buka, and B. Welch, "Smoking Habits of High School Students in Newton, Massachusetts," *The New England Journal of Medicine* 265 (1961): 969–974.

3. E. J. Salber and J. Worcester, "Change in Women's Smoking Patterns," *Cancer* 17 (1964): 32–36.

4. E. J. Salber and M. Feinlieb, "Breast-Feeding in Boston," *Pediatrics* 37 (1966): 299–303.

5. E. J. Salber, D. Trichopoulos, and B. MacMahon, "Lactation and Reproductive Histories of Breast Cancer Patients in Boston, 1965–66," *Journal of the National Cancer Institute* 43 (1969):1013–1024.

6. W. Zinsser, *On Writing Well: An Informal Guide to Writing Nonfiction* (New York: Harper & Row, 1980), p. 131.

Transition

1. No woman held a tenured position at Harvard Medical School until the mid-1960s. P. A. Norbert, "Women Firsts at Harvard: Student and Faculty Pioneers," in *Women at Harvard: The First 350 Years* (Cambridge, Mass., Radcliffe Quarterly, 1986), p. 8.

2. For an encyclopedic history of Boston in the sixties and seventies, see J. A. Lukas, *Common Ground: A Turbulent Decade in the Lives of Three American Families* (New York: Alfred A. Knopf, 1985).

The Bracken Field Health Center

1. The passage of twenty years frees me to tell that the real name of the health center I directed is the Martha Eliot Family Health Center. But because I wrote a book about the center shortly after my resignation, I called it by a different name: The Bracken Field Health Center. The names of the people I write about in this chapter are the same as those I gave them in that book. For the sake of consistency I am keeping to the old names here.

2. M. Harrington, *The Other America: Poverty in the United States* (Baltimore: Penguin Books, 1973).

3. The Federal Office of Economic Opportunity, better known as OEO, funneled this grant money to its Boston branch: Action for Boston Community Development. The *local* antipoverty unit most closely connected with the health center was the West Hill Area Planning Action Committee, known as APAC.

4. L. Lawson, *Working Women: A Portrait of South Africa's Black Women Workers* (Braamfontein: Ravan Press, 1985), p. 17.

5. K. B. Clark, *Dark Ghetto: Dilemmas of Social Power* (New York and Evanston, Ill.: Harper & Row, 1965), p. xv.

6. E. J. Salber, J. J. Feldman, H. Offenbacher, and S. Williams, "Characteristics of Patients Registered for Service at a Neighborhood Health Center," *American Journal of Public Health* 60 (1970): 2273–2283.
7. E. J. Salber, J. J. Feldman, L. A. Rosenberg, and S. Williams, "Utilization of Services at a Neighborhood Health Center," *Pediatrics* 47 (1971): 415–423.
8. E. J. Salber, J. J. Feldman, H. Johnson, and E. McKenna, "Health Practices and Attitudes of Consumers at a Neighborhood Health Center," *Inquiry* 9 (1972): 55–61.
9. P. H. Wise, M. Kottelchuck, M. Wilson, and M. Mills, "Racial and Socioeconomic Disparities in Childhood Mortality in Boston," *The New England Journal of Medicine* 313 (1985): 360–366.
10. E. J. Salber, "Community Participation in Neighborhood Health Centers," *The New England Journal of Medicine* 283 (1970): 515–518.
11. E. J. Salber, *Caring and Curing: Community Participation in Health Services* (New York: Neale Watson Academic Publications, 1975).

Moving South: A New Beginning

1. For two excellent comparative histories of racism and segregation in South Africa and the United States see: G. M. Fredrickson, *White Supremacy: A Comparative Study in American & South African History* (New York: Oxford University Press, 1981) and J. W. Cell, *The Highest Stage of White Supremacy: The Origins of Segregation in South Africa and the American South* (New York: Cambridge University Press, 1982).
2. T. L. Beyle and M. Black, eds., *Politics and Policy in North Carolina* (New York: MSS Information Corporation 1975), pp. 1–3.
3. U.S. Department of Health, Education, and Welfare Public Health Services, *Health United States 1975* (Rockville, Maryland: National Center for Health Statistics 1975), pp. 225, 347, 354, 355.
4. Mary Mebane reported that at her black university campus, black professors and administrators favored light-skinned students over those at the "black black" end of the scale. M. Mebane, *Mary* (New York: Viking Press, 1981), pp. 208–216.
5. B. Head, Foreword to E. Kuzwayo, *Call Me Woman* (San Francisco: Spinsters Ink, 1985), p. xiii.

Settling Down at Duke

1. D. Tutu, "Foreword" in *South Africa: The Cordoned Heart: Essays by Twenty South African Photographers*, ed. O. Badsha (Cape Town: Gallery Press, 1986) p. xiv and (New York and London: W. W. Norton, 1986).

2 Health Planning Council for Central North Carolina, *Durham Health Care for the 70's: A Report on the Health Care Needs of Durham* (Durham, N.C., 1973).

3. My staff and I maintained close ties with the health advisory board members, visited them in their homes, set up a health education program for them, and consulted with them on our community activities. In turn they were extraordinarily helpful to us.

4. For an enlightening and lively account of the life and work of a revenue agent who pursued men and women making and selling illicit liquor in North Carolina, see: A. Wilkinson, *Moonshine: A Life in Pursuit of White Liquor* (New York: Penguin Books 1986).

5. E. J. Salber, S. B. Greene, J. J. Feldman and G. Hunter, "Access to Health Care in a Southern Rural Community" *Medical Care* 14 (1976): 971–986.

6. S. B. Thacker, E. J. Salber, C. Osborne and L. H. Muhlbaier, "Primary Care in Durham County: Who Gives Care to Whom?" *Medical Care* 17 (1979): 69–78.

7. S. B. Thacker, E. J. Salber, C. Osborne and L. H. Muhlbaier, "Primary Care in an Academic Medical Center" *American Journal of Public Health* 68 (1978): 853–857.

8. D. E. Walls, *The Chickenbone Special* (New York: Harcourt Brace Jovanovich, 1971).

*Health Facilitators: Lay Advisers
in Community Health*

1. T. Ferguson, "Taking Care of Each Other," *Medical Self-Care* (Winter 1982), pp. 16–21.

2. The names and positions of senior staff, office staff, coordinators, facilitators, and volunteer resource persons all appear in one or other of our publications describing this program.

3. E. J. Salber, W. Beery, and E. Jackson, "The Role of the Health Facilitator in Community Health Education," *Journal of Community Health* 2 (1976): 5–20. C. Service and E. J. Salber, eds., *"Community Health Education: The Lay Advisor Approach"* (Durham, Duke University Department of Community and Family Medicine, 1977). E. J. Salber, "The Lay Advisor as a Community Health Resource," *Journal of Health Politics, Policy and Law* 3 (1979): 469–478. E. J. Salber, "Where Does Primary Care Begin? The Health Facilitator as a Central Figure in Primary Care," *Israel Journal of Medical Sciences* 17 (1981): 100–111.

4. At the completion of our first training program, I interviewed each of the participants in their homes in order to gauge their understanding of the program and their satisfaction with it.

Don't Send Me Flowers When I'm Dead

1. E. J. Salber, *Don't Send Me Flowers When I'm Dead: Voices of Rural Elderly* (Durham: Duke University Press, 1983).
2. I changed the names of the people I interviewed and the area in which they lived because some members of their families feared strangers knowing the whereabouts of their defenseless parents.
3. E. J. Salber, *Caring and Curing: Community Participation in Health Services* (New York: Neale Watson Academic Publications, 1975).
4. Dr. Dominic D'Eustachio and Dr. Duncan Heron took the photographs, thirty of which appear in the book.
5. E. J. Salber, S. B. Greene, J. J. Feldman, and G. Hunter, "Access to Health Care in a Southern Rural Community," *Medical Care* 14 (1976): 971–86.
6. S. S. Hill, *Religion and the Solid South* (New York: Abingdon Press, 1972), pp. 24–56.

Photo Credits

Ken Gooch, University of Cape Town 4
© Elizabeth van Ryssen, University of Cape Town 19
Catharine Carter, from a painting by P. W. Lamb 25
Ferdie Stern 63
Eva J. Salber 65
© *The Cape Argus*, Cape Town 73
Harry T. Phillips 96
Durban City Health Department, Durban 97
Harry T. Phillips 100
Ken Gooch, University of Cape Town 110
Zwelethu Mthethwa 111
Stan Schubert, University of Cape Town 120
© *The Cape Argus*, Cape Town 127
Kathleen Crampton 173
Kathleen Crampton 175
Theresa Carsten 186
Kathleen Crampton 191
Theresa Carsten 201
Kathleen Crampton 203
Program staff 243
© Dominic D'Eustachio 254
Duncan Heron 258
© Dominic D'Eustachio 260
© Dominic D'Eustachio 263
Duncan Heron 265
Duncan Heron 266
Duncan Heron 269
Joseph Thomas, *The News and Observer*, Raleigh 272
Sheila Borsook 273

Library of Congress Cataloging-in-Publication Data
Salber, Eva J.
The mind is not the heart.

Bibliography: p.
Includes index.
   1. Salber, Eva J.   2. Women physicians—United States
—Biography.   3. Women physicians—South Africa—Biog-
raphy.   I. Title.
R154.S215A3   1989   610'.92'4 [B]   88-33557
ISBN 0-8223-0910-6